Access supplemental video content online at MediaCenter.Thieme.com!

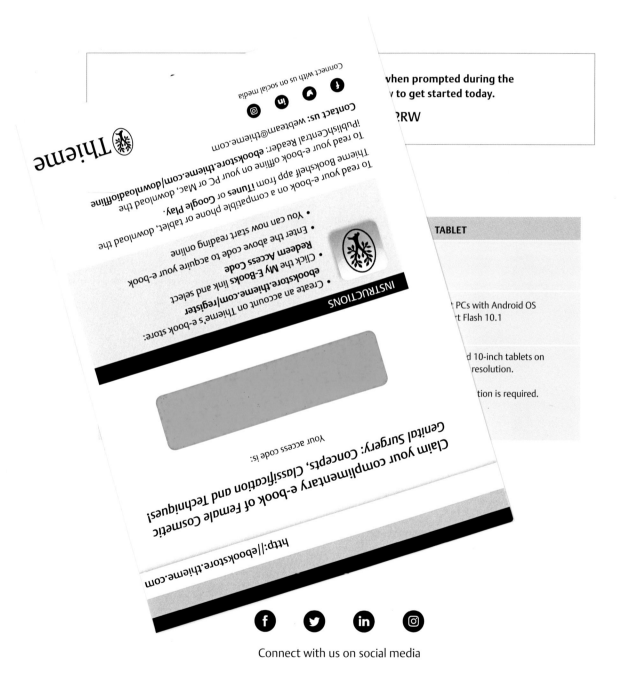

INSTRUCTIONS

Create an account on Thieme's e-book store:
eBookstore.thieme.com/register

- Click the **My E-Books** link and select
Redeem Access Code
- Enter the above code to acquire your e-book
- You can now start reading online

To read your e-book on a compatible phone or tablet, download the Thieme Bookshelf app from **iTunes** or **Google Play**.

To read your e-book offline on your PC or Mac, download the iPublishCentral Reader: **eBookstore.thieme.com/downloadOffline**

Contact us: webteam@thieme.com

Connect with us on social media

Thieme

Your access code is:

Claim your complimentary e-book of Female Cosmetic Genital Surgery: Concepts, Classification and Techniques!

http://ebookstore.thieme.com

TABLET

...PCs with Android OS
...rt Flash 10.1

...d 10-inch tablets on
...resolution.

...tion is required.

...when prompted during the
...y to get started today.

...?RW

Connect with us on social media

Female
Cosmetic
Genital Surgery

Concepts, Classification, and Techniques

Female
Cosmetic
Genital Surgery

Concepts, Classification, and Techniques

Edited by

Christine A. Hamori, MD, FACS
Board-Certified Plastic Surgeon
Founder and Director, Cosmetic Surgery and Skin Spa
Boston, Massachusetts

**Paul E. Banwell, BSc(Hons), MB BS,
FRCS(Eng), FRCS(Plast)**
Consultant Plastic, Reconstructive and Aesthetic Surgeon
The Banwell Clinic
The McIndoe Centre
East Grinstead, West Sussex, United Kingdom

Red Alinsod, MD, FACOG, FACS
Director, South Coast Urogynecology and
Alinsod Institute for Aesthetic Vulvovaginal Surgery
Laguna Beach, California

With Illustrations by
Brenda L. Bunch, MAMS
Amanda Yarberry Behr, MA, CMI
Craig Durant, Dragonfly Media
Andrea Hines

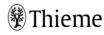 Thieme

Executive Editor: Sue Hodgson
Managing Editor: Haley Paskalides
Developmental Editor: Jennifer Gann
Project Managers: Becky Sweeney and Suzanne Wakefield
Director, Editorial Services: Mary Jo Casey
Production Editors: Torsten Scheihagen and Naamah Schwartz
International Production Director: Andreas Schabert
International Marketing Director: Fiona Henderson
International Sales Director: Louisa Turrell
Director of Sales, North America: Mike Roseman
Senior Vice President and Chief Operating Officer: Sarah Vanderbilt
President: Brian D. Scanlan

Library of Congress Cataloging-in-Publication Data

Names: Hamori, Christine A., editor. | Banwell, P. (Paul E.), editor. | Alinsod, Red, editor.

Title: Female cosmetic genital surgery : concepts, classification, and techniques / [edited by] Christine A. Hamori, Paul E. Banwell, Red Alinsod.

Description: New York : Thieme, [2017] | Includes bibliographical references.

Identifiers: LCCN 2016050534 (print) | LCCN 2016051532 (ebook) | ISBN 9781626236493 (print) | ISBN 9781626237711 (ebook)

Subjects: | MESH: Gynecologic Surgical Procedures--methods | Genitalia, Female--surgery | Reconstructive Surgical Procedures--psychology

Classification: LCC RG104 (print) | LCC RG104 (ebook) | NLM WP 660 | DDC 618.1/059--dc23

LC record available at https://lccn.loc.gov/2016050534

©2017 Thieme Medical Publishers, Inc.

Thieme Publishers New York
333 Seventh Avenue, New York, NY 10001 USA
+1 800 782 3488, customerservice@thieme.com

Thieme Publishers Stuttgart
Rüdigerstrasse 14, 70469 Stuttgart, Germany
+49 [0]711 8931 421, customerservice@thieme.de

Thieme Publishers Delhi
A-12, Second Floor, Sector-2, Noida-201301
Uttar Pradesh, India
+91 120 45 566 00, customerservice@thieme.in

Thieme Publishers Rio de Janeiro, Thieme Publicações Ltda.
Edifício Rodolpho de Paoli, 25° andar
Av. Nilo Peçanha, 50 – Sala 2508,
Rio de Janeiro 20020-906 Brasil
+55 21 3172-2297 / +55 21 3172-1896

Cover design: Thieme Publishing Group
Typesetting by Elaine Kitsis, Debra Clark

Printed in China by Everbest   5 4 3 2 1

ISBN 9781626236493

Also available as an ebook:
eISBN 9781626237711

Important note: Medicine is an ever-changing science undergoing continual development. Research and clinical experience are continually expanding our knowledge, in particular our knowledge of proper treatment and drug therapy. Insofar as this book mentions any dosage or application, readers may rest assured that the authors, editors, and publishers have made every effort to ensure that such references are in accordance with **the state of knowledge at the time of production of the book.**

Nevertheless, this does not involve, imply, or express any guarantee or responsibility on the part of the publishers in respect to any dosage instructions and forms of applications stated in the book. **Every user is requested to examine carefully** the manufacturers' leaflets accompanying each drug and to check, if necessary in consultation with a physician or specialist, whether the dosage schedules mentioned therein or the contraindications stated by the manufacturers differ from the statements made in the present book. Such examination is particularly important with drugs that are either rarely used or have been newly released on the market. Every dosage schedule or every form of application used is entirely at the user's own risk and responsibility. The authors and publishers request every user to report to the publishers any discrepancies or inaccuracies noticed. If errors in this work are found after publication, errata will be posted at www.thieme.com on the product description page.

Some of the product names, patents, and registered designs referred to in this book are in fact registered trademarks or proprietary names even though specific reference to this fact is not always made in the text. Therefore, the appearance of a name without designation as proprietary is not to be construed as a representation by the publisher that it is in the public domain.

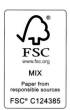

DEDICATION

To my Mom and Dad

Christine A. Hamori

To Jo, Seb, Belle, and Enzo

Paul E. Banwell

This book is dedicated with affection to my Mom and Dad, Nap and Erlinda, who gave me my foundation in life and love for God. My wife, Robyn, and children, Samantha, Dillon, Matthew, and James, who are my sources of warmth each and every day. My brother Arr and sister DG, who have stuck by my side with laughter and vigor. And to my office staff team of Diane, Maria, Marisol, Cindy, and Eunice—it is you who have brought cheer and laughter to my every day.

Red Alinsod

CONTRIBUTORS

Red Alinsod, MD, FACOG, FACS
Director, South Coast Urogynecology
and Alinsod Institute for Aesthetic
Vulvovaginal Surgery, Laguna Beach,
California

**Paul E. Banwell, BSc(Hons), MB BS,
FRCS(Eng), FRCS(Plast)**
Consultant Plastic, Reconstructive and
Aesthetic Surgeon, The Banwell Clinic,
The McIndoe Centre, East Grinstead,
West Sussex, United Kingdom

Nicolas Berreni, MD
Surgical Gynecologist and Obstetrician,
Genital Restoration Center, Karis
Institut, Perpignan, France; Researcher,
Medical Imaging Department,
ENSEEIHT Polytechnic School,
Toulouse, France

Christine A. Hamori, MD, FACS
Board-Certified Plastic Surgeon; Founder
and Director, Cosmetic Surgery and Skin
Spa, Boston, Massachusetts

Kharen Ichino
Premedical Student, University of Texas
at Austin, Texas; Medical Assistant to
Dr. Jennifer L. Walden, Private Practice
of Dr. Jennifer L. Walden, Austin, Texas

Evgenii Leshunov, MD
Department of Urology and
Andrology, Russian Medical Academy
of Postgraduate Study; Scientific
Coordinator, Association of Gender
Medicine, Moscow, Russia

**Colin C.M. Moore, FRCS, FRACS,
FACCS, FAMLC**
Associate Professor, Faculty of Medicine,
Monash University, Melbourne, Victoria,
Australia; Associate Professor, Director of
Surgery, Australian Centre for Cosmetic
Surgery, Sydney, New South Wales,
Australia

**Marco A. Pelosi II, MD, FACS, FACOG,
FICS, FAACS**
Director, Pelosi Medical Center,
Bayonne, New Jersey

Marco A. Pelosi III, MD
Chairman, Obstetrics and Gynecology,
International College of Surgeons–
United States Section; Associate Director,
Pelosi Medical Center, Bayonne, New
Jersey

Otto J. Placik, MD, FACS
Assistant Professor of Clinical Surgery–
Plastic, Department of Surgery,
Northwestern University Feinberg School
of Medicine, Chicago, Illinois

Neal R. Reisman, MD, JD, FACS
Clinical Professor, Department of Plastic
Surgery, Baylor College of Medicine;
Chief, Department of Plastic Surgery,
CHI Baylor St. Luke's Medical Center,
Houston, Texas

Charles Runels, MD
American Cosmetic Cellular Medicine
Association, Fairhope, Alabama

Clara Santos, MD
Medical Doctor, Department of
Dermatology, Red Cross Hospital, São
Paulo, São Paulo, Brazil

Lina Triana, MD
Plastic Surgeon, Clinica Corpus y
Rostrum, Cali, Valle, Colombia

Jennifer L. Walden, MD, FACS
Owner and Medical Director, Jennifer
L. Walden, MD, PLLC and Walden
Cosmetic Surgery and Laser Center,
Austin, Texas

FOREWORD

I am delighted to have been asked to write a foreword for this new book, *Female Cosmetic Genital Surgery: Concepts, Classification, and Techniques,* which provides essential guidance for surgeons who perform genital rejuvenation procedures for their female patients. I warmly congratulate Dr. Hamori, her co-editors, and all contributors for this comprehensive, beautiful, much-needed, and timely contribution to our medical literature.

The first description of a purely aesthetic form of labiaplasty, provided by Drs. Darryl Hodgkinson and Glen Hait, appeared in a medical journal more than 30 years ago (*Plastic and Reconstructive Surgery,* 1984). According to statistics from the American Society for Aesthetic Plastic Surgery, nearly 9000 patients underwent labiaplasty procedures in the United States in 2015, representing a 16% increase from 2014 to 2015. These statistics are for labiaplasty alone and do not include associated procedures such as vaginal tightening. In 2015, given the rapid growth and demand for genital rejuvenation, combined with the need for valid peer-reviewed information, the *Aesthetic Surgery Journal* added a Genital Rejuvenation Section in recognition of the importance of these procedures.

Indications for the procedures are both physical and psychosocial. Studies have already appeared in the literature validating the effectiveness of genital rejuvenation in meeting physical and psychosocial needs of patients seeking such treatments.

Continuing demand and growth in these procedures makes the timing of Dr. Hamori's book particularly appropriate. The contents have been carefully assembled and cover essential topics such as informed consent, psychosocial issues, and "what is normal anatomy," before a discussion of the different surgical options, from the standard curved linear resection and wedge procedures, to hymenoplasty, to innovations such as treatment with fat grafts and fillers, representing a wealth of experience of surgeons worldwide. There is a chapter devoted to avoidance and management of complications. The Advances section explores developing treatments such as radiofrequency and fractionated lasers. The book is well written and beautifully and liberally illustrated with specially designed artwork. Well-produced, clear, instructional video presentations of the key surgical procedures accompany many chapters. All of the content can be accessed online as well as in the more traditional print format.

This comprehensive new book is an invaluable resource to surgeons worldwide who aim to help women seeking these procedures by operating on them safely to achieve the best possible outcomes. I am confident this will be the "go to" source for genital rejuvenation and have great pleasure in recommending it.

Foad Nahai, MD, FACS, FRCS
Maurice J. Jurkiewicz Chair in Plastic Surgery
    and Professor of Surgery
Department of Surgery
Emory University
Atlanta, Georgia

FOREWORD

It is an honour for me to be invited to write a foreword for *Female Cosmetic Genital Surgery: Concepts, Classification, and Techniques.* Drs. Christine Hamori, Paul Banwell, and Red Alinsod have compiled a comprehensive volume which examines the various techniques of aesthetic and functional female genital surgery. Chapters dealing with the psychosocial issues and informed consent are most welcome in this relatively new and developing area of body contour surgery.

Knowledge of the perineal anatomy is, of course, essential to any practitioner who is contemplating a surgical approach to the female genital area. Paul Banwell has reviewed this topic thoroughly, and his review of the morbid anatomy probably represents the first time most plastic surgeons will have encountered this area since their anatomy class back in medical school. The exception to this being surgeons who perform inner thighplasty, which also requires a background to the important vascular and neurological features of the female genital area. In addition to knowing the anatomy, it is imperative that the surgeon also appreciates the aesthetic goals of the patient.

When Glen Hait and I wrote our review of labiaplasty (*Plastic and Reconstructive Surgery,* 1984), we could not have foreseen that the procedure would have become so widely accepted and adopted by so many of our colleagues within just a few decades. At that time, the surgery was not seen as it is today—as an aesthetic procedure—thus our paper also reviewed female circumcision, discussing the sociological, religious, and historical traditions of that procedure.

Whether the ever-growing acceptance of female genital procedures by surgeons in the last 30 years has been fueled by the increase in demand or vice versa, what is certain is that any taboos regarding female genital surgery no longer exist in many parts of the world. Social trends and the acceptability of nudity in the media, especially on the Internet, encourage women to seek aesthetic genital surgery to improve their self- and sexual image. The desire to feel more feminine and in many cases wear more-tight-fitting clothing and swimwear is a prime motivating factor in seeking consultation.

Back in 1983 things were different, and the patients who presented had symptoms relating to discomfort and hygiene. At that time, I was working in Tidewater, Virginia, which is extremely humid in summer, making hygiene an issue for many women with large labia minora. Dr. Hait, who was from Arizona, helped patients who predominantly complained of discomfort when sitting in a saddle while riding horses. Both of our patient groups were predominantly presenting with functional problems. Now, three decades later in an era when Brazilian waxing and pubic hair modification is commonplace, there is much more awareness of the shapes and forms of female genitalia in general and of the possibility for its surgical modification.

Female Cosmetic Genital Surgery: Concepts, Classification, and Techniques is both a timely and well-structured book that presents the updated techniques used by major contributors to the literature. Long-term satisfaction with various trimming, tailoring, and augmenting techniques is reviewed in detail. As technology has advanced for our nonsurgical options in so many areas of rejuvenation of the face and body, so too has technology contributed to a new era of vaginal rejuvenation.

The future of female genital surgery is assured, and this landmark textbook will be of great value to all surgeons prepared to work with their female patients to achieve both functional and aesthetically pleasing results.

Darryl J. Hodgkinson, MB BS(Hons), FACS,
    FRCS(C) plastic surgery, FACCS
Private Practice
Sydney, Australia

PREFACE

"All truth passes through three stages. First, it is ridiculed. Second, it is violently opposed. Third, it is accepted as being self-evident."

—Arthur Schopenhauer

During the late 1990s, when I was fresh out of my plastic surgery residency, I met a young woman who requested a reduction of her labia minora. She felt uncomfortable in her clothes and was embarrassed to be intimate. My first thought was that she must have a body dysmorphic disorder. Why would someone want to alter an area concealed by hair and that was primarily functional? After I examined her, I understood her concern. Her labia minora were large and protrusive, and this was accentuated by the fact that she had very little pubic hair.

I agreed to perform a labiaplasty, and I fully disclosed to the patient that this would be the first time I had performed such a surgery. She consented, and I searched the literature for guidance. There only existed a small paragraph on the procedure in McCarthy's *Plastic Surgery,* as well as a handful of case reports about severe hypertrophy of the labia. In 1998, just as I was about to perform this procedure, Gary Alter (a plastic surgeon trained in urology) published his wedge resection technique for the reduction of hypertrophic labia minora.

I performed the wedge resection with the assistance of a urology colleague. The patient did well and returned years later professing her gratitude for my performance of this life-enhancing procedure. She now wanted a breast augmentation. This experience helped me to realize how important genital appearance is to women, so I did not shy away from helping them to enhance this area. More women presented to me with labial hypertrophy, and I became more proficient in its treatment. However, this taboo procedure was slow to gain traction in the plastic surgery community.

One would expect that, as the popularity of labiaplasty increased, scientific due process would precede aggressive marketing. Unfortunately, gynecologic pioneers in the field engaged in the promotion of niche procedures and extolled the benefits of "laser vaginal rejuvenation." In 2007, a statement was released by the American College of Obstetrics and Gynecology questioning such procedures due to the paucity of evidence-based research supporting its safety and benefits. Again, in light of this statement, the validity of the field of female aesthetic surgery was questioned.

Over the next decade, my diverse practice grew, as did my interest in and experience with aesthetic vaginal surgery. Much to the chagrin of my old-school European father, I began to lecture and publish in this area, and I was labeled an expert in the field. The physiological and psychological benefits of labiaplasty were discovered and published in plastic surgery peer-reviewed journals. Surgical series demonstrated high patient satisfaction and low complication rates.

Fast forward another decade, and I now have more than 400 labiaplasties under my belt (forgive the pun), driven in part by a shift toward nude pubic grooming. I was delighted when I was approached by the publisher to write a book about female cosmetic genital surgery. I feel that the field is finally approaching validation in the plastic surgery community. Together with the help of plastic surgeons, gynecologists, and urologists, I have been able to create a comprehensive resource for the field of female aesthetic vaginal surgery. Our book covers, first, principles, including a detailed chapter on anatomy and the important topic of consent issues. This is followed by stepwise guidance for the performance of different procedures, including more than 350 color photographs and beautiful, bespoke surgical illustrations. To further aid understanding, the book includes more than 10 fully narrated video clips showing details of surgery. Finally, the book is available in both print and electronic formats, so it can be accessed easily wherever the reader may be. It is my hope that young specialists going into this growing field will find this book an inspiration to further expand the specialty.

Christine A. Hamori

ACKNOWLEDGMENTS

I wish to thank Jean Sidoti for her endless support in finding time for me to create this book.

Christine A. Hamori

I would like to thank my family, teachers, students, and friends for their inspiration and loyal support over the years. Special mention goes to Professor Michael Morykwas and Richard Parker, Esq. Great leaders. Great minds and great friends.

Last, and most important, I would like to thank Jo, Seb, Belle, and Enzo. Love and laughter never die. You are my reason for being.

Paul E. Banwell

This book would not be possible without the vision of Giants. First, thank you David Matlock for the many arrows you took on our behalf. Thank you to the Pelosis for their organizational and surgical brilliance, to Team Miklos and Moore for their passion and dedication to our "new" field, and to Michael Goodman, Christine Hamori, and Paul Banwell for friendships strengthened by fire. Last, to my loyal friend from Day 1, Otto Placik. You always make me look good.

Red Alinsod

CONTENTS

VIDEO CONTENTS

Part I
Introduction

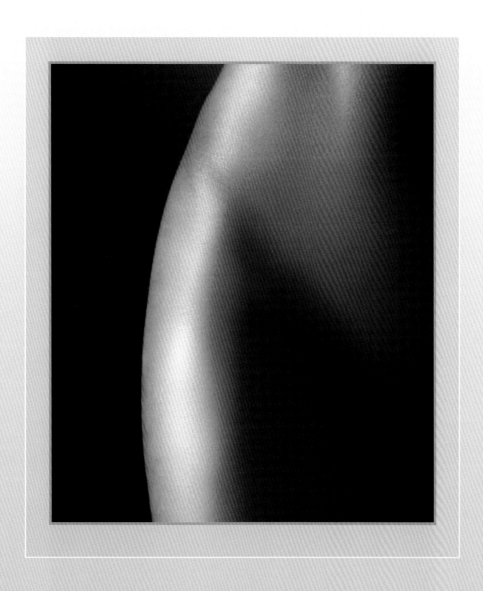

Anatomy and Classification of the Female Genitalia: Implications for Surgical Management

Paul E. Banwell

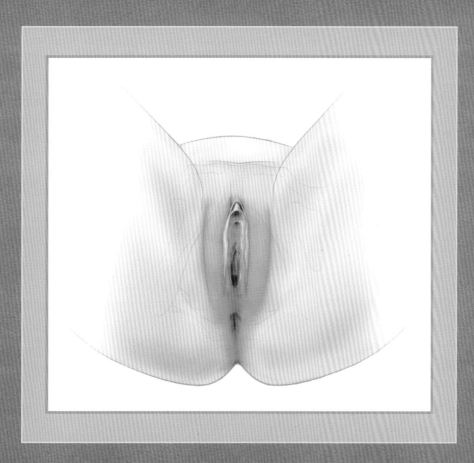

Key Points

- *Understanding the anatomy of the female genitalia is fundamental to surgical planning and technique in cosmetic surgery of this area.*

- *Systematic examination of the mons, labia majora, clitoris, and labia minora (vulval complex) is essential.*

- *Wide variations exist in the anatomy of the vulval complex.*

- *Hodgkinson and Hait's aesthetic ideal of small labia minora not protruding beyond the labia minora are a desired goal of most patients.[1]*

- *In parallel with facial aesthetics and facial harmony, surgeons should consider the concept of genital harmony.*

- *Newly documented insights into the vascular anatomy of this area may influence choice of technique.*

- *The Motakef classification[2] describes the degree of labia minora protrusion beyond the labia majora.*

- *The Banwell classification[3] describes variations in the shape and morphology of the labial anatomy that have not been previously documented.*

- *The clitoral hood–labia minora complex in particular varies widely in appearance and is potentially a problematic area for surgeons.*

- *Careful documentation of the size and shape of the labia and the labial-clitoral complex (according to Motakef and Banwell) is critical.*

As the popularity of female genital surgery in our practices rises, we have seen a parallel increase in published clinical experience, available operative techniques, and mounting data in the scientific literature espousing the physical and non-physical benefits of such procedures. As shall be explored further in this book, we now have strong evidence for high patient satisfaction, minimal complication rates, and excellent safety profiles, as well as published evidence on the psychological benefits. However, to date there have been few attempts to classify the female external genitalia, a paucity of information on common anatomic variants, and little exploration or re-evaluation of the anatomy in relation to operative techniques, surgical planning, and treatment outcomes.

A sound understanding of current anatomy and knowledge of previously unrecognized anatomic variations within the female genitalia may therefore help surgeons optimize a tailored approach and offer new insights into patient care.

Applied Anatomy for Surgeons

The anatomy of the external female genitalia has been well described[4] (Fig. 1-1). It consists of the mons pubis superiorly (venus mont), the clitoris with its overlying clitoral hood, the labia majora, and the labia minora. Collectively, most anatomic texts refer to this as the *vulval complex.* However, much of the variation in the anatomic arrangement has not been previously recognized or described; awareness and understanding of these variations may be particularly pertinent to surgical planning.[5]

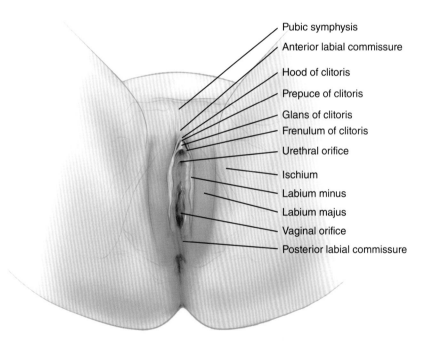

Pubic symphysis
Anterior labial commissure

Hood of clitoris
Prepuce of clitoris
Glans of clitoris
Frenulum of clitoris
Urethral orifice
Ischium
Labium minus
Labium majus
Vaginal orifice
Posterior labial commissure

Fig. 1-1 Basic gross anatomy of the female external genitalia.

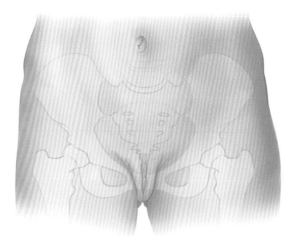

Fig. 1-2 The relationship between a youthful mons and the pubic rami.

Mons Pubis

The mons pubis is a triangular adipose tissue elevation situated anterior to the pubic symphysis (Fig. 1-2). This adipose tissue can increase during puberty or with weight gain, but it also lessens with significant weight loss and after menopause. The mons pubis is anatomically covered by pubic hair, which also decreases with age during the perimenopausal period. The prominence of the mons area can vary enormously not only because of increased fat deposition but also because of the angle of the pubic rami; both are reasons for presentation for surgical reduction of this area.

Labia Majora

The labia majora (outer lips) are two cutaneous folds that extend posteriorly from the mons pubis toward the perineal region (Fig. 1-3). They have a hair-bearing outer (lateral) aspect and an inner aspect that lacks hair. Each labia majora is filled with subcutaneous fibrofatty tissue to varying degrees but can vary from "full" and "tight" to "lax" and "baggy," as patients often describe (Fig. 1-4). Our common practice, however, is to document a lax and baggy appearance as "empty" or "redundant" tissues.

Enveloped (to varying degrees) and medial to the labia majora are the clitoris and clitoral hood and the labia minora. The labia majora are usually separated from the labia minora by a deep sulcus; this is typically well-defined and a useful surgical boundary between non-hair-bearing and hair-bearing skin (Fig. 1-5). Rarely, the deep, subcutaneous vertical attachments of this sulcus are tenuous or even absent, leading to a less-defined continuum between the labia majora and minora. In such cases, if a labia majora reduction is considered, then the scar may potentially become more visible, and this should be discussed in detail with the patient preoperatively.

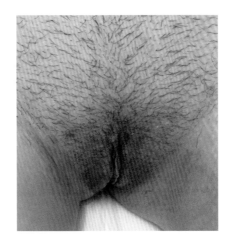

Fig. 1-3   Youthful labia majora.

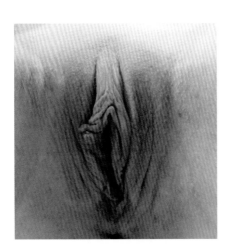

Fig. 1-4   Empty labia majora, commonly described by patients as "baggy." The skin is redundant and empty. This patient presented for labia majora reduction and revision surgery of the labia minora. The original procedure was performed elsewhere.

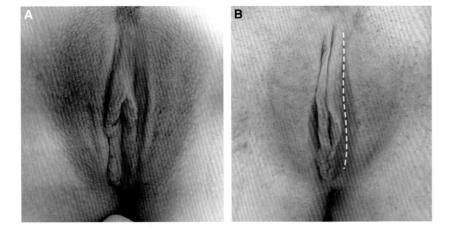

Fig. 1-5   A, This patient was referred for labia majora reduction and revision of the labia minora surgery performed previously by a colleague. The tissue pigmentation is not uncommon. **B,** Hair-bearing skin and non-hair-bearing skin. The *dotted line* represents the labia majora sulcus and the boundary between hair-bearing and non-hair-bearing skin. This is a useful surgical landmark for the medial marking for labia majora reduction (see Chapter 6: Labia Majora Reduction Surgery: Majoraplasty).

The Clitoris

The clitoris (clitoral body) superiorly is located under a clitoral hood (prepuce) that splits into a frenulum on either side of the introitus (vaginal vault) (Fig. 1-6). According to classic anatomic texts, the frenulum attaches most commonly to the outer aspect of the upper third of the labia minora (Fig. 1-6, *A*), but as seen throughout this book and as explored in more detail later in the chapter, this arrangement varies widely. The clitoral body itself can also vary significantly in size, and usually a larger clitoral body is associated with heavier clitoral hood skin. A second fold of skin may be present lateral to the clitoral hood, which either fuses with the labia minora (Fig. 1-6, *G* and *H*) or remains dominant and in continuity with the labia minora (Fig. 1-6, *I*). Last, at the apex of the frenulum, the urethral meatus can usually be found.

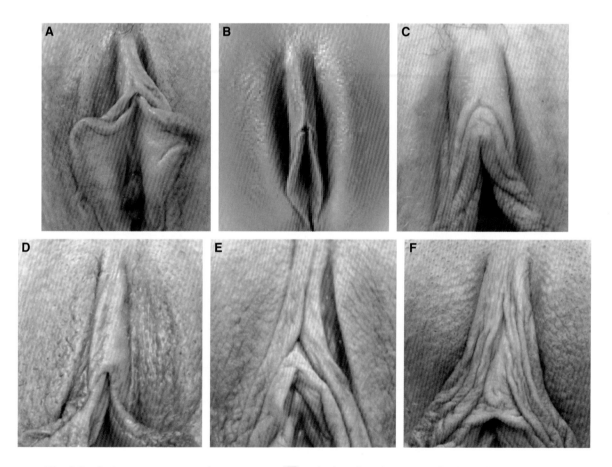

Fig. 1-6   A, A common anatomic arrangement seen in the clitoral area, as displayed in most classic anatomic texts. The clitoral hood and the superior aspect of the labia minora fuse together. The variation in this junction has implications for clinical outcomes and patient expectations and should be considered when choosing a surgical technique. **B,** A small clitoral hood continuous with the labia minora. **C,** A heavy clitoral hood. **D,** A small clitoral hood. The frenulum is continuous with the labia minora. The right side demonstrates small lateral fold. **E,** A lateral clitoral double fold. **F,** Multiple lateral clitoral folds.

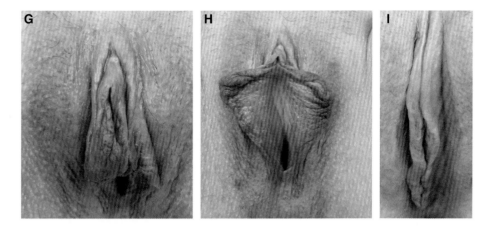

Fig. 1-6, cont'd   G and **H,** A double clitoral fold inserting into the lateral aspect of the labia minora. **I,** A lateral double fold that is dominant and continuous with the labia minora. The clitoral body and clitoral hood are hidden.

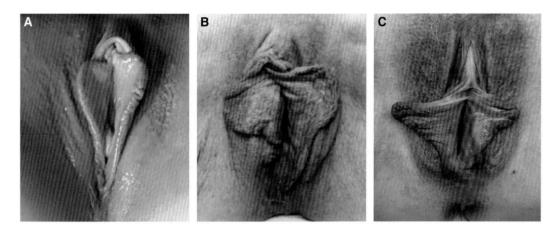

Fig. 1-7   A, Small, firm labia minora. **B,** Loose, rugose labia minora. **C,** Asymmetry within the labia minora. The lateral edge has loose, rugose tissues and pigmentation.

Labia Minora

The labia minora continue posteriorly from the clitoral area toward the perineal body either joining to form the posterior fourchette or remaining separate and attaching to the perineum (Fig. 1-7). The appearance and shape of the labia minora have many variations; asymmetries are extremely common, and clinicians specializing in female genital surgery soon become aware that the anatomic variation may be very diverse. Furthermore, the skin quality may vary. Surgeons will note that some patients have youthful and tight labia (see Fig. 1-7, *A*), but usually, patients presenting for this operation have tissues that are very loose and rugose in nature (Fig. 1-7, *B*). Often pigmentation is noted. Some of the more common variations of labia minora morphology will be discussed later in the chapter.

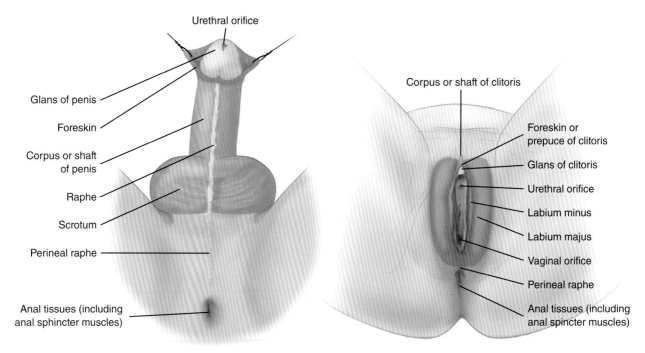

Fig. 1-8   The labia majora are analogous to the scrotum. The labia minora become fused in males (perineal raphe). Wolffian ducts develop in males, and Müllerian ducts develop in females. Differences develop at approximately 9 weeks' gestation. In the female, a deep groove forms around the phallus. The sides of it grow dorsalward as the labioscrotal folds, which ultimately form the labia majora in females. The labia minora, in contrast, arise by the continued growth of the lips of the groove on the undersurface of the phallus; the rest of the phallus forms the clitoris. The immature glans becomes the clitoral glans. In the male, the pelvic portion of the cloaca undergoes much greater development, pushing before it the phallic portion. The labioscrotal folds extend around and between the pelvic portion and the anus and form a scrotal area. During the changes associated with the descent of the testes, this scrotal area is drawn out to form the scrotal sacs. The penis is developed from the phallus. As in the female, the urogenital membrane undergoes absorption, forming a channel on the undersurface of the phallus; this channel extends only as far forward as the corona glandis.

Embryology

Embryologically, the labia majora in women are derived from the genital swellings that, in the male fetus, develop into the scrotum (Fig. 1-8). In contrast, the labia minora develop from the genital folds, which, in the male fetus, fuse to form the median raphe.

Blood Supply

The blood supply to the labia minora and majora consists of the posterior labial artery and the perineal artery, both branches of the internal pudendal artery. Similarly, the internal pudendal artery, deep to the perineal membrane, also gives rise to the dorsal artery of the clitoris.

However, Georgiou et al[6] provided additional detailed insight into the vascular anatomy of the labia minora based on their recent cadaveric arterial injection study. They also provided thoughts on the choice of technique for labia minora reduction: They suggested that the main complication of the different surgical reduction techniques is dehiscence of the suture line, and that the vascular anatomy may not always be respected, especially, perhaps, with flap techniques (Fig. 1-9). In the study, they identified a dominant central artery (C artery), two posterior arteries (P1 and P2), and one small anterior artery (A) (Fig. 1-10). They confirmed a connection between the anterior system of the external pudendal artery and the posterior system of the internal pudendal artery. They concluded that this may help surgeons with orientation of wedge excisions. Their anatomic study also confirmed that the curvilinear excision method is the safest with the most robust blood supply.

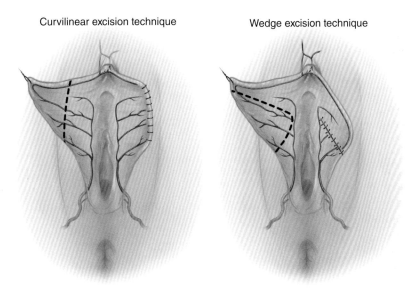

Fig. 1-9   The blood supply in relation to curvilinear and wedge excision techniques.

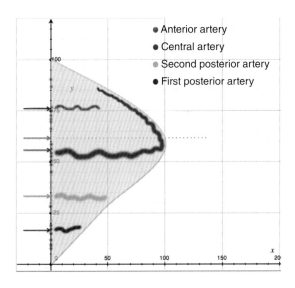

Fig. 1-10   Mapping of the labial arteries demonstrating the A, C, and P arteries.

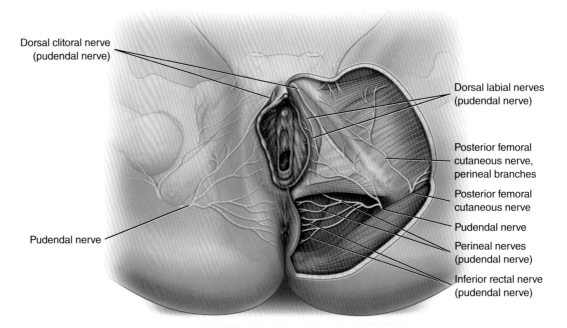

Dorsal clitoral nerve
(pudendal nerve)

Dorsal labial nerves
(pudendal nerve)

Posterior femoral
cutaneous nerve,
perineal branches

Posterior femoral
cutaneous nerve

Pudendal nerve

Perineal nerves
(pudendal nerve)

Inferior rectal nerve
(pudendal nerve)

Pudendal nerve

Fig. 1-11   The pudendal and dorsal nerve of the clitoris.

Nerve Supply

The innervation to the external female genitalia is through the pudendal nerve (Fig. 1-11). This splits at the superficial transverse perineal muscle into the superficial and deep perineal nerves. The superficial branch becomes the posterior labial nerve, and the deep branch becomes the dorsal nerve of the clitoris.

Classifications of Female Genital Anatomy

According to Lloyd et al,[7] the genital dimensions in women vary considerably; thus the spectrum of normality is wide. In their observational, cross-sectional study, they measured a variety of parameters, including labial length and width, clitoral size and color, and rugosity of the labial skin. They noted a wide range of values for each measurement (up to 5 cm for labial width), and they found no statistically significant association with age, parity, ethnicity, hormone use, or history of sexual activity. This point is important,

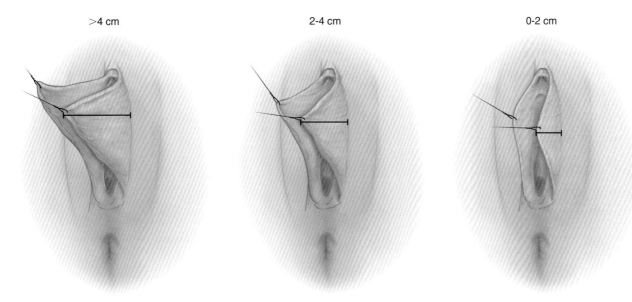

>4 cm   2-4 cm   0-2 cm

Fig. 1-12 Motakef classification for labial protrusion, which classifies the degree of protrusion of the labia minora past the labia majora. Class I (0 to 2 cm), class II (2 to 4 cm), and class III (more than 4 cm) may be amenable to different treatment paradigms. An "A" is added for asymmetry and a "C" for involvement of the clitoral hood.

because it is vital for surgeons to reassure patients who wish their genitalia to be surgically modified that their genitalia are well within normal limits.

A few authors have documented their approach to the assessment of labia (minora) projection, but there is no consensus as to how to best classify the appearance of the female genitalia. Motakef et al[2] have recently performed a meta-analysis of labiaplasty publications and highlighted the paucity of information for practicing surgeons regarding a suitable classification (Fig. 1-12). We talk about labial "hypertrophy" and "enlargement," but some patients with labia of "normal" size still desire a more sculpted appearance.

One of the most widely used classification systems, first described by Franco and Franco[8] in 1993, classifies labial hypertrophy into four types: type I, less than 2 cm; type II, 2 to 4 cm; type III, 4 to 6 cm; and type IV, more than 6 cm. The authors measured the distance (in centimeters) from the base of the labia minora (the vaginal introitus) to the outermost labial point. They too found that labia minora vary in length, thickness, symmetry, and protuberance. In another study, the mean width of the labia minora was found to be 2.5 cm, with a range of 0.7 to 5 cm.[9]

In contrast, Chang et al[10] suggested a simplified classification based on the size and location of the genital protrusion. Class 1 is normal anatomy; the labia majora and minora are about equal. In class 2, the labia minora protrude beyond the labia majora. In class 3, a clitoral hood is present. In class 4, large labia minora extend to the perineum. The authors suggested that different classes should be approached using different techniques.

More recently, Motakef et al[2] have proposed an elegant classification system for labial protrusion based on the distance of the lateral edge of the labia minora from that of the labia majora rather than from the introitus. According to their system, labial protrusion may therefore be classified as class I (0 to 2 cm), class II (2 to 4 cm), or class III (more than 4 cm) (see Fig. 1-13).

Our group concurs with this approach and has evolved similar thoughts over the last 10 years based on results of measuring from the lateral sulcus to the most prominent point. Perhaps most important, Motakef et al[2] also indicated that different classes of labial protrusion may be amenable to different treatment paradigms—a tailored approach to labial reduction using different methods must therefore be considered. This philosophy is further supported by the vascular anatomic studies described previously.[6]

We have also found that adopting an objective approach and measuring (and documenting) the labial dimensions helps when discussing the degree of reduction desired by the patient. Rather than using more nebulous words such as *sculpted* or *neat* or discussing *overcorrection* or *undercorrection,* a more objective approach involving percentages can be adopted. Performing more than or less than a 50% reduction therefore becomes fairly straightforward, because this can be accurately measured in preoperative marking and facilitates discussions regarding expected outcomes.[11] As documentation in aesthetic surgery becomes evermore important, not only from a medicolegal perspective but also in aiding treatment strategies, we encourage all surgeons to document the appearance and size of the labia. Reconstructive and cosmetic surgeons pay particular attention to measurements and pre-existing appearances when planning cosmetic breast surgery, for example, and labiaplasty requires the same degree of attention.

Documentation and Classification of Anatomic Variants

The Banwell classification of labial anatomy[5] has been developed to account for the previously unrecognized anatomic presentations that surgeons may encounter when consulting with prospective patients requesting labial reduction. This has helped to educate patients, aid in surgical planning, and facilitate discussions among medical colleagues.

Essentially, the scheme documents the specific anatomic appearance and arrangement of the labia minora and perineal takeoff. It also takes into account any double-fold arrangement of the frenulum between the clitoris and the labia minora. We think documentation of these anatomic variations and measurements of the labia should be required of all clinicians.

Labia Minora Morphology

Variations in the shape of the labia minora should be noted (Fig. 1-13). Conveniently, prominence of the most lateral point in the labia minora may occur in the upper, middle, or lower third of the vaginal vault. These are classified as type I, type II, and type III, respectively. The consistency and rugosity of the labia should be noted, along with pigmentation.

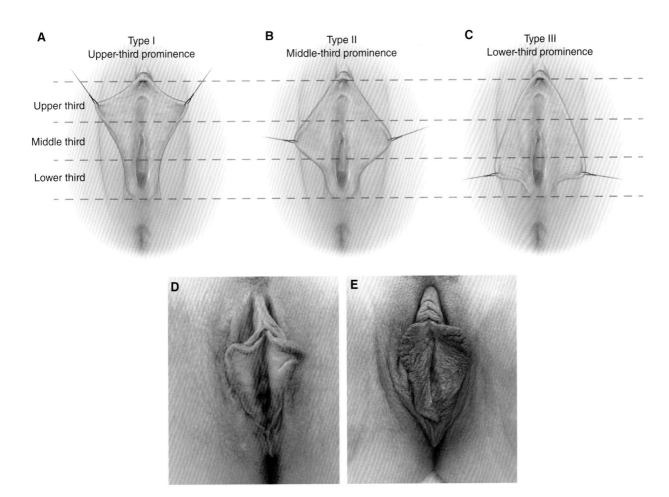

Fig. 1-13 Banwell classification of labia minora morphology. **A,** Type I: Upper-third enlargement (winging). **B,** Type II: Middle-third enlargement. **C,** Type III: Lower-third enlargement. **D,** The most common arrangement is type I with upper-third prominence. **E,** Type I: Upper-third enlargement. The pigmentation within the labia should be noted and pointed out to patients, because it has implications for matching up edges when using the wedge technique (see Chapter 4: Labial Reduction: Surgical Wedge Technique).

Labial asymmetry

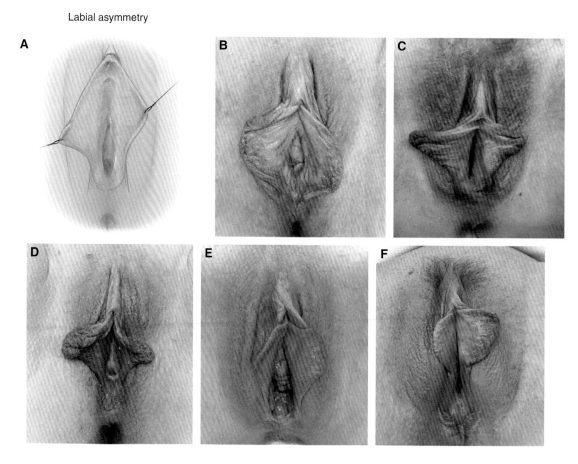

Fig. 1-14   A, Banwell classification of labial symmetry and asymmetry. **B,** Type II (middle third on the right) and type III (lower third) on the left associated with pigmentation. **C,** Type I (upper third) enlargement with asymmetry (right greater than left). **D,** Type I asymmetry, left; type II asymmetry, right (right greater than left). **E,** Labial asymmetry type II (middle third bilaterally), but the left is greater than the right. **F,** Type II asymmetry (left greater than right).

Labial Symmetry and Asymmetry

Labial asymmetry is extremely common and, as with other cosmetic surgery (for example, of the breasts and ears), should be documented carefully and pointed out to patients (Fig. 1-14). Asymmetries may occur in the absolute dimensions of the same anatomic variation, or asymmetries may involve different anatomic variations.

Labial Perineal Takeoff

The posterior attachments of the labia minora also vary, and this is designated "labial perineal takeoff." As with labial morphology, this also had implications for surgical planning (Figs. 1-15 and 1-16). They are conveniently divided into low (closest to the perineum), medium, and high. Examples of each are shown below. Some patients with a low perineal takeoff may also have a connected posterior fourchette, which is particularly pertinent with wedge techniques (see Chapter 4: Labial Reduction: Surgical Wedge Technique).

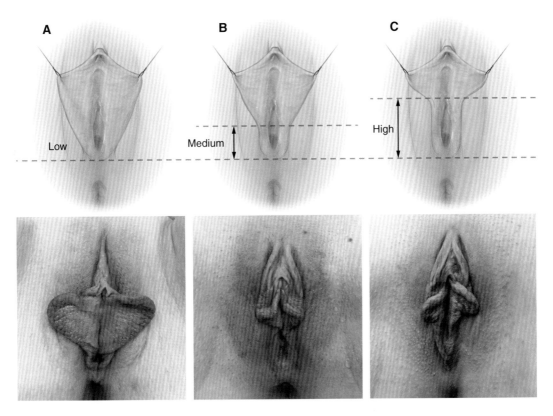

Fig. 1-15 The labia minora perineal takeoff. **A,** Low takeoff. **B,** Medium takeoff. **C,** High takeoff.

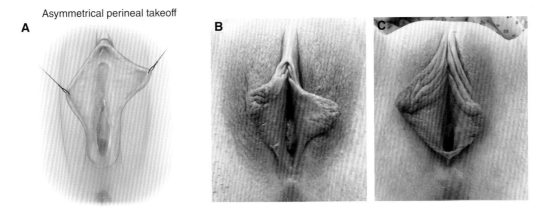

Fig. 1-16 **A,** Asymmetrical perineal takeoff. A woman could have both asymmetrical labial enlargement and an asymmetrical perineal takeoff. **B,** Labial asymmetry in dimension, morphology, and perineal takeoff: Type I (upper third) on the right and type II (middle third) on the left. The perineal takeoff is also asymmetrical. **C,** Type II (middle third) enlargement on the right, type III (lower third) enlargement on the left, and a triple clitoral fold. This patient also has a connected posterior fourchette, which is important to note in wedge techniques.

Clitoral-Labial Complex

Not surprisingly, the clitoral-labial complex is also subject to significant size and anatomic variations. In traditional anatomic texts the clitoral body and hood are small but both may be noted to be hyperplasic and even disproportionate to the labia. Usually a bilateral frenulum radiates from a small clitoral hood and inserts into the posterior aspect of the labia minora (Fig. 1-17).

In other patients, we have noted the clitoral hood itself is almost vestigial, and a *lateral* clitoral double-fold arrangement may be present. In these situations, the lateral clitoral skin creates a more significant double-fold arrangement and will fuse variably with the labia minora. This usually creates a labial-dominant or a clitoral-dominant pattern (Fig. 1-18). Variations on this theme are shown in Fig. 1-19 and should be noted carefully, because this may influence choice of surgical technique.

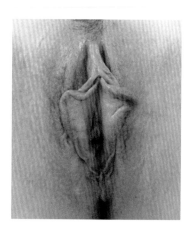

Fig. 1-17   The traditionally known arrangement with a small hood and frenulum inserting into the posterior aspect of the labia minora.

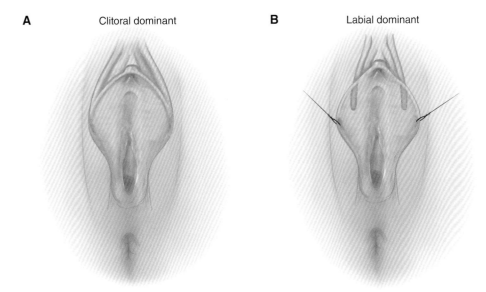

Fig. 1-18 Anatomy of the clitoral double fold. Highlighting and documenting such anatomic arrangements are critical. **A,** Clitoral dominance. The appearance in keeping with traditional anatomic texts. The frenulum of the clitoris fuses with the labia minora to create a double fold. **B,** Labial dominance with a double fold that is clitoral-hood dominant. The labia minora have a vestigial origin.

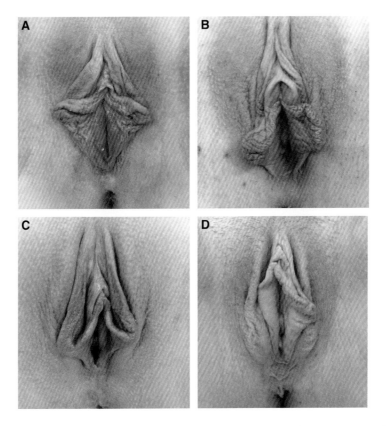

Fig. 1-19 **A,** Type I (upper third) enlargement with a lateral double-fold arrangement (clitoral dominance). The clitoral hood is almost vestigial. **B,** Type II (middle third) enlargement, lateral clitoral double fold with labial dominance. **C,** Type II (middle third) enlargement. This is a very rare arrangement with a double fold and equal labial and clitoral dominance. **D,** Type II asymmetry, left; type I asymmetry, right (left greater than right). A double fold with labial dominance.

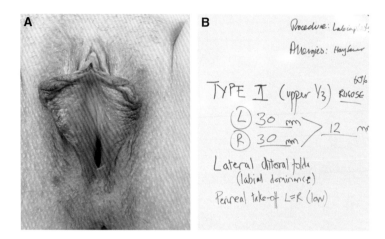

Fig. 1-20   A, Intraoperative anatomic findings. **B,** The findings as noted in the operating room by the surgeon.

Documentation of the Anatomy

As part of our normal practice, we note our clinical findings intraoperatively and document them on the surgery board and in the operative note. As shown in Fig. 1-20, the labial morphology has been confirmed (type I), together with the presence of a lateral clitoral fold, the perineal takeoff, and the rugose nature of the tissues. The dimensions of the labia minora were noted (according to Motakef) in millimeters. Preoperatively, the patient and surgeon agreed to a percentage reduction of 60%, and this was measured and marked accordingly.

Aesthetic Ideals

The concept of *aesthetic ideals* has gained increasing traction recently with specific reference to the ideal shape of the breast.[12] Parallels have been made in other areas of cosmetic surgery. Currently, there is no established aesthetic ideal regarding the appearance of the labia minora, although in the first description of aesthetic labiaplasty technique, Hodgkinson and Hait,[1] in their seminal paper, suggested that labia minora protruding past the labia majora are perhaps both aesthetically and functionally unsatisfactory.

Supporting this concept, Hamori[13,14] and others have cogently argued that social trends have influenced our concepts of aesthetic ideals. The ubiquity of Brazilian waxing, models in the media clad in sheer clothing with no labial show, and the anonymity of internet pornography may contribute to a new standard of vulval beauty. In addition to the labia minora, the labia majora has been scrutinized in favor of a smooth and full profile.

Furthermore, Placik and Arkins[15] examined Playboy magazine centerfold photography and suggested a subtle shift and trend toward the visibility and prominence of the female genitalia as the focal point of popular nude photographs rather than the breasts.

Although an increasing number of patients desire these evolving ideals and features, they are not universally accepted goals. Ensuring our patients have realistic expectations is essential; we cannot promise these appearances will be achieved in every patient because of the huge variation of anatomic presentations, as seen in this chapter. Therefore, in a drive toward tailoring treatment for our patients, the concept of *genital harmony* (or proportion) as a more desired goal, within the context of an individual's anatomy, is emerging. Perhaps this term implies a more measured approach, involving discussions about balance and harmony (as in the facial aesthetic arena) rather than about trying to achieve an aesthetic ideal.

Conclusion

Surgeons undertaking female genital surgery should understand that the vulval complex has wide anatomic variations. These have been recognized and incorporated into new classification systems. The size and shape of the genitalia should be considered very carefully when choosing the appropriate surgical technique; we recommend procedures are therefore individualized according to anatomy.

The concept of aesthetic ideals is evolving; however, surgical outcomes should aim for genital harmony within the context of a patient's anatomy. Last, and perhaps most important, we propose that an objective approach with careful documentation and measurement of the external genitalia should be required for surgeons performing female cosmetic genital surgery.

References

1. Hodgkinson DJ, Hait G. Aesthetic vaginal labioplasty. Plast Reconstr Surg 74:414, 1984.
2. Motakef S, Rodriguez-Feliz J, Chung MT, et al. Vaginal labiaplasty: current practices and a simplified classification system for labial protrusion. Plast Reconstr Surg 135:774, 2015.
3. Banwell PE. Classification and anatomical variations of the female genitalia: implications for labiaplasty surgery. J Plast Reconstr Aesthetic Surg (submitted for publication).
4. Standring S, ed. Gray's Anatomy: The Anatomical Basis of Clinical Practice, ed 41. Philadelphia: Elsevier, 2016.
5. Banwell PE. Labiaplasty: anatomy, techniques and new classification. Clinical Cosmetic & Reconstructive Expo, Olympia, London, Oct 2013.
6. Georgiou CA, Benatar M, Dumas P, et al. A cadaveric study of the arterial blood supply of the labia minora. Plast Reconstr Surg 136:167, 2015.
7. Lloyd J, Crouch NS, Minto CL, et al. Female genital appearance: "normality" unfolds. BJOG 112:643, 2005.

8. Franco T, Franco D. Hipertrofia de ninfas. J Bras Ginecol 103:163, 1993.

9. Dobbeleir JM, Landuyt KV, Monstrey SJ. Aesthetic surgery of the female genitalia. Semin Plast Surg 25:130, 2011.

10. Chang P, Salisbury MA, Narsete T, et al. Vaginal labiaplasty: defense of the simple "clip and snip" and a new classification system. Aesthetic Plast Surg 37:887, 2013.

11. Banwell PE. Latest advances in labiaplasty: ideas and ideals. Keynote address. Cosmetex, Melbourne, Australia, Apr 2013.

12. Mallucci P, Branford OA. Population analysis of the perfect breast: a morphometric analysis. Plast Reconstr Surg 134:436, 2014.

13. Hamori CA. Aesthetic surgery of the female genitalia: labiaplasty and beyond. Plast Reconstr Surg 134:661, 2014.

14. Hamori CA. Discussion: Vaginal labiaplasty: current practices and a simplified classification system for labial protrusion. Plast Reconstr Surg 135:789, 2015.

15. Placik OJ, Arkins JP. Plastic surgery trends parallel Playboy magazine: the pudenda preoccupation. Aesthet Surg J 34:1083, 2014.

CHAPTER 2

Psychological Issues and Social Mores in Female Genital Aesthetic Surgery: What Is Normal?

Kharen Ichino, Jennifer L. Walden

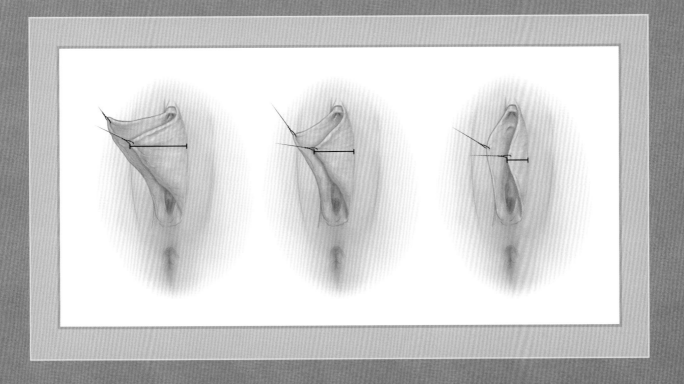

Key Points

- *No consensus exists regarding what constitutes a normal external appearance of the female genitalia.*

- *The contemporary Western ideal of the "perfect vagina" is often described as hairless and pink with labia minora not projecting beyond the labia majora.[1]*

- *Studies show a wide range of sizes for each part of the genitalia, making it difficult to describe normal measurements.[2]*

- *Psychological improvements are well described in women who have undergone female aesthetic surgical genital procedures for cosmetic and functional reasons.[3,4]*

- *The highly controversial topic of female genital mutilation (FGM) or female genital cutting (FGC)—excising parts of the female genitals for traditional or religious beliefs—is still practiced in third world countries and is their norm of female genital beauty.[5]*

- *The beauty norm is completely subjective for each patient and should help to improve psychological, physical, and sexual states, even in cases of aesthetic genital surgery.*

As with technology and fashion, the perceptions of beauty are constantly evolving. Well into the 1950s, aesthetic plastic surgery occurred in secret and was considered a taboo subject to even mention.[6] Today, because of the organization of national plastic surgical societies around the world, millions of cosmetic surgery procedures have been performed. For instance, the American Society for Aesthetic Plastic Surgery (ASAPS), consisting of experienced and well-qualified aesthetic plastic surgeons, has published data suggesting that approximately 16 million cosmetic surgeries were performed in the United States in 2014.[7] The most popular procedures such as breast augmentation and liposuction are familiar to many and have paralleled the definitions of modern beauty. Labiaplasty, which has been performed since the late 1970s,[3] is increasing rapidly in number. Women are not yet as comfortable discussing this procedure openly despite the increase in awareness across all media channels. According to ASAPS, (Cosmetic Surgery National Data Bank Statistics), 8745 women had labiaplasty (excluding vaginal rejuvenation) in 2015 in the United States.[8] This number may seem small compared with the other popular procedures mentioned, but it has increased by 44% from 2013—evidence of a trend that will probably continue to rise significantly[9] (P. Banwell, personal communication, 2016).

The increasing desire for labiaplasty worldwide begs a few questions: Is there such thing as a "perfect" vagina, and what is considered normal? This chapter addresses the different cultural definitions of female genital beauty and the wide variants of normal. Not only the physical but also the psychological improvements that aesthetic genital surgery can provide will be discussed, as well as the associations and implications of FGM on contemporary society.

The Rise in Labiaplasty: Social Influences

The rise in demand of labiaplasty for aesthetic and functional reasons has increased significantly in Western culture. Labiaplasty has been practiced since the 1970s, when, even then, women thought that the labia minora should not protrude beyond the labia majora for aesthetic and functional satisfaction.[3] The gradual increase in this trend is suspected to result from the ease in access of images and information through the Internet, such as the perfectly bare vaginas seen in pornography and photoshopped pictures of celebrities in tight-fitting clothes, lingerie, and swimwear. Snug-fitting clothes like leggings and yoga pants have become fashion trends that lead women to be more cautious about the way their crotch is contoured.[10] Sex talk is more prominent among liberated young women, but their genitals are rarely discussed in detail. Unlike men, even when women are completely naked in front of other women, genital details are usually not exposed. This ambiguity prevents many women from becoming aware of all the size, shape, and color variations; thus images seen in pornography and textbooks are referred to as *normal*.

In some studies, most women described a pretty vagina to be hairless and pink with the labia minora very small or nonexistent.[1] In a recent documentary written by Lisa Rogers entitled "The Perfect Vagina,"[1] women as young as 16 years of age were concerned with the way their vagina looked. A 16-year-old girl thought that her boyfriend would not be attracted to her after seeing her genitalia, so she decided to have surgery at a relatively early age. In another case, a 21-year-old woman was teased by her own sister for having a "hangy" and verbally teased by her male friends who had never even seen it themselves. She was too embarrassed to present herself in front of medical professionals, so she neglected going to her annual gynecology examinations, which could have led to more serious health problems. In these two cases, views of the opposite sex played a role, yet cultural studies showed that 98% of heterosexual men never care about the appearance of a vagina, in contradiction to what modern Internet pornography leads many to think.[10] Despite the indifference of the opposite sex, some women self-critique by comparing themselves to the images of perfect vaginas.

The Western View

In countries such as United States, the United Kingdom, and Australia, where cultural and religious views are diverse, female genital beauty ideals are very subjective. Sex education and the function of genitalia are taught in school, but young women usually are not informed in much detail about the variety of sizes, shapes, and colors. The lack of this information leads many young girls to wonder if the external appearance of their vagina is normal. Lloyd et al[2] conducted a study in 2004 to answer this question. They measured different parts of the vagina—including the clitoris, labia majora, and labia minora—and the variation of colors of 50 different women who ranged in age from 18 to 50 years and were of different ethnicities. Overall, the women described an ideal vagina as having all parts small. However, the results showed that the clitoral size ranged from 5 to 35 mm, the labia majora length 7 to 12 cm, the labia minora length 20 to 100 mm, and the labia minora width 7 to 50 mm. These ranges were too wide to determine a trend for normal vaginal measurements. Even in medical literature, few descriptions are given of a normal, external appearance of female genitalia, probably because there is no normal. Whether the labia minora are visible when a woman is standing is a subjective matter. Most consider the female genitalia to be adequate and normal if it functions properly. To further emphasize that normal genitals come in all appearances, artist Jamie McCartney from the United Kingdom created a wall sculpture made with plaster casts of 400 different women's genitals, which has been displayed at Triennale Museum in Milan, London Mall Galleries, and other exhibits.[11]

Sharp et al[12] found, in one of the first published qualitative studies involving labiaplasty patients, findings that suggested that online media and negative peer commentary played an important role in women's decisions to undergo labiaplasty. Women are usually satisfied with the results of their labiaplasty and therefore in their psychological and sexual well-being. However, women's expectations in their sexual relationships were not always fulfilled, as might be expected.

The Non-Western View

As opposed to the liberal attitudes in countries previously mentioned, where many undergo genital procedures for functional or aesthetic reasons, Southeast Asia and many parts of Africa have standard, completely different cultural norms for female genitalia. In these areas of the world, religious reasons are given for conducting genital procedures.

FGM or FGC is considered highly controversial and illegal in Western societies.[5] Many women in third world countries live in extremely religious and/or traditional communities where everything that the community does is done together and not questioned. Many Muslims who follow the teachings in the Koran believe that excising parts of their labia, clitoral hood, or even the whole clitoris is a sign of purity and more desirable in a wife.

Young girls usually are not given a choice to have this procedure but do so because it is the normal thing to do. Often, girls are not informed that they will undergo an excision but instead are taken away to have a painful and unexpected procedure. Women of these communities who had FGM and were asked if they knew the reason for this process all answered "no," but, because everyone had undergone the procedure, they perceived it as normal and asked no questions.[5]

The idea of having surgery without a reason or choice is far from comprehensible for many westernized people who have complete authority over what is done to their own body. As many Westerners think, nonprotruding labia minora define genital beauty, whereas women who undergo FGM think this alteration defines beauty. The spectrum of what makes female genitalia normal is broad; therefore how this most intimate body part is treated and its appearance are each woman's decision. No matter what others say, perspective about oneself should be a priority.

Psychological Ramifications of Female Genital Aesthetic Surgery

Psychological improvements have been noted in women who personally chose to have vaginal rejuvenative procedures, and, by contrast, in those who had FGM without choice.[5,13] Of 258 women who underwent a procedure for aesthetic reasons, approximately 92% were satisfied with the results.[13] Sexual satisfaction, although a subjective assessment, significantly increased in women and their partner. This may have resulted from the psychological effect of knowing that surgery was completed rather than from sensation, given that surgery affects sensory cutaneous nerves. Others noted positive cosmetic effects not related to function or sexual intercourse. The 21-year-old discussed previously, who was teased by her sister, reported that she was satisfied with herself as soon as her labia were surgically trimmed. Despite the inevitable postoperative discomfort and pain, she explained how life changing the procedure was.[1] Although none of her male friends who teased her had seen her genitals preoperatively, and studies showed that most heterosexual males do not take notice of the appearance of genitals,[10] she gained self-confidence. As with any type of aesthetic surgical procedure on any part of the human anatomy, this subjective self-image can be life changing no matter how differently others perceive it.

Female Genital Mutilation and Cultural Values

FGM has been a controversial topic discussed for decades and banned in modernized countries, yet these rituals still take place in nonwesternized rural areas such as Africa and Southeast Asia.[14] Women who went through the process all said they were in pain but not in fear and were "very happy" when they had it done.[5] Acceptance from their community and family overpowered fear and pain. Fear can be the main driving force of certain human actions, and for them, the main fear was disappointing their family and community, which outweighed their physical pain. In such communities, having FGM is a must and less stressful than questioning the ways of ancestors. Many of these women questioned people who did not go through this ritual and considered them a disgrace.[5]

Infibulation is a type of FGM in which most of a woman's clitoris, labia minora, and at times labia majora are excised and the vulva sutured closed in a way that covers the vagina except for a small hole that allows menstrual blood and urine to escape. This is an extreme measure to ensure chastity in which only in the presence of the husband can the vagina be reopened for sexual intercourse, and it is stitched back up in his absence. It is traditional in some Northeastern African cultures but also highly controversial. It is an act of oppression to women, who are born to be wives and conceive as many children as they can. Without any personal freedoms, including freedom to work, their sole purposes are to satisfy their husband and be accepted by the community. In this regard, the procedure is a sign of being a great wife and a guarantee of matrimonial loyalty. Many people are in disbelief of this practice and think that it is irrational; however, from the perspective of community members, those who are not mutilated are considered odd. It very much goes against most Western mores, yet to those cultures, the women are able and determined to pass on this ritual to their daughters. In such a community with extremely homogeneous views, trying to alter them may cause more trauma and unwanted tension among the people.[14]

Similarly, young women in some Middle Eastern cultures voluntarily seek hymenoplasty. Because some religions strictly require young women to be virgins until marriage, the women who have already had sexual relations decide to have their hymen repaired. The hymen is a membrane that partially or completely covers the vaginal opening. Most people think this is what tears during their first intercourse and describe it as their "cherry being popped."[13] A Muslim girl, for example, wanted to have her hymen repaired before her arranged marriage, because she knew she would be shunned by her family if they found out that she was not a virgin.[1] She stated that her parents would rather kill themselves than have it known to others that their daughter lost her virginity before marriage. When interviewed on their thoughts of marrying a girl who had lost her virginity before marriage, men and women of the same religion replied that it was unacceptable under any circumstances.[1] The repulsion from the opposite sex and the belief that death is a better prospect than losing virginity before marriage causes serious stress and tension among women in this culture. Many westernized people may oppose this girl's decision, but for her, having it repaired meant psychological relief. These young Muslim women seek a procedure that they think will benefit their life in their community, regardless of whether the decision conflicts with personal views.

Core Differences Between Aesthetic Genital Surgery and Female Genital Mutilation

Four ethical principles distinguish FGM from aesthetic genital surgery: (1) the autonomy of the patient, (2) nonmaleficence, (3) beneficence, and (4) justice.[13] These principles help to ensure that patients wishing to undergo the procedure do so by choice with a well-qualified surgeon, with support in a noncoercive manner, and with appropriate, informed consent. FGM is traditionally performed without notice or consultation, whereas with westernized aesthetic genital procedures, the proposed operation, its risks, benefits, potential complications, and postoperative care are discussed in detail preoperatively.

Conclusion

Whether there is a norm for external female genitalia is in question, but many patients have psychological improvements after female genital aesthetic surgery.[4] Because of the wide range of measurements for each part of the genitalia, determining specific, *normal* measurements is difficult. This variability and constant access to its imagery in contemporary society explain why aesthetic surgery of the female genitalia is rising in popularity, and why labiaplasty surgery itself provides an overall high patient satisfaction.[3,4] Psychology and sexual medicine literature have established a correlation between the levels of comfort women have with the intimate areas of their body and how they positively affected sexual functions.[3,15] After this type of surgery, women report an improvement in body perception, sexual confidence, and overall sex life with a decrease in discomfort.

References

1. Leach H. (Director), Rogers L. (Writer). The Perfect Vagina [Video file]. Top Documentary Films. Available at *http://topdocumentaryfilms.com/perfect-vagina/*.

2. Lloyd J, Crouch NS, Minto CL, et al. Female genital appearance: "normality" unfolds. BJOG 112:643, 2005.

3. Hamori CA. Aesthetic surgery of the female genitalia: labiaplasty and beyond. Plast Reconstr Surg 134:661, 2014.

4. Miklos JR, Moore RD, Chinthakanan O. Overall patient satisfaction scores, including sexual function, following labiaplasty surgery: a prospective study comparing women with a history of prior cosmetic surgery to those with none. Plast Reconstr Surg 134:124, 2014.

5. Walker A, Parmar P. Warrior Marks: Female Genital Mutilation and the Sexual Blinding of Women. San Diego: Harcourt Brace, 1993.

6. American Society of Plastic Surgeons. American Society of Plastic Surgeons reports cosmetic procedures increased 3 percent in 2014. Available at *http://www.plasticsurgery.org/news/2015/plastic-surgery-statistics-show-new-consumer-trends.html*.

7. American Society for Aesthetic Plastic Surgery. Press Center. ASAPS looks back on 35 years of cosmetic surgery. Available at *http://www.surgery.org/media/news-releases/asaps-looks-back-on-35-years-of-cosmetic-surgery*.

8. American Society for Aesthetic Plastic Surgery. Cosmetic Surgery National Data Bank Statistics, 2015. Available at *http://www.surgery.org/sites/default/files/Stats2015.pdf*.

9. American Society for Aesthetic Plastic Surgery. Press Center. Statistics, Surveys, & Trends. Labiaplasty and buttock augmentation show marked increase in popularity. Available at *http://www.surgery.org/media/news-releases/labiaplasty-and-buttock-augmentation-show-marked-increase-in-popularity*.

10. Holloway K. The labiaplasty boom: why are women desperate for the perfect vagina? Alternet. Available at *http://www.alternet.org/news-amp-politics/labiaplasty-boom-why-are-women-desperate-perfect-vagina*.

11. McCartney J. The Great Wall of Vagina. Available at *http://www.jamiemccartney.com/main/works/C9*.

12. Sharp JM, Mattiske J, Vale KI. Motivations, expectations, and experiences of labiaplasty: a qualitative study. Aesthetic Surg J 2016 Feb 23. [Epub ahead of print]

13. Dobbeleir JM, Landuyt KV, Monstrey SJ, et al. Aesthetic surgery of the female genitalia. Semin Plast Surg 25:130, 2011.

14. Amnesty International. Infibulation in Africa. Available at *http://www.witchhazel.it/female_genital_mutilation.htm*.

15. Goodman M, ed. Sexual and psychological ramifications. In Goodman M, ed. Everything You Ever Wanted to Know About Women's Genital Plastic & Cosmetic Surgery. Pressbooks.com, 2013. Available at *http://drgoodman.pressbooks.com/chapter/chapter-3sexual-and-psychological-ramifications/*.

CHAPTER 3

Informed Consent and Liability in Cosmetic Genital Surgery

Neal R. Reisman

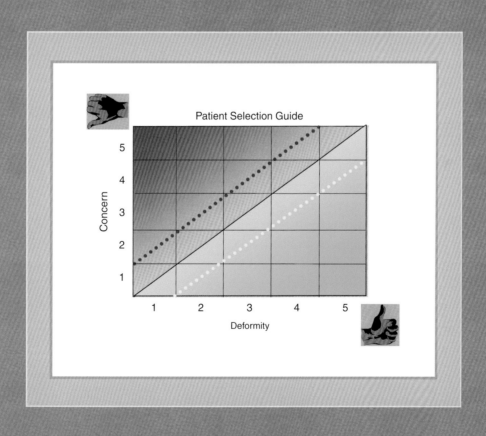

Key Points

- *Appropriate patient expectations are essential.*

- *Patient goals should be realistic for the procedure.*

- *Informed consent is a process, NOT the signed paper.*

- *Surgeons should be honest in their disclosure about the effects of new procedures.*

Basic Medicolegal Issues

The basic medicolegal issues include elements of a tort, informed consent, the definition of *damages,* and specific financial and warranty issues. Most female patients seeking aesthetic surgery of their genitalia do so electively. This has an impact on tort law, which establishes four elements for a tort claim:

- A duty to treat the patient
- A breach of that duty
- Proximate cause
- Damages

The first element to establish in a medical negligence claim is a duty to treat the patient. This duty may begin once a patient is accepted into the practice. Therefore realistic expectations and appropriate timing for surgery are essential. The second element is a breach of that duty. This may include what has been described as the *battle of the experts.* A standard of care is defined with difficulty and suggests the appropriate level of care that a reasonable physician would use to treat a patient. A standard of care comprises many methods, all of which are acceptable, although different physicians might select different methods. When choosing procedures and a treatment plan, it is always helpful to consider peer-accepted procedures. If a new procedure or method is contemplated, it should be fully discussed with the prospective patient so that it is not perceived as experimenting in a new area. The third element, proximate cause, establishes that the breach of action or inaction is directly responsible for damages. This is also known as the "but for" element in that *but for* the action or inaction, damages would not have occurred. The last element is damages. This can be confusing for physicians in that complications of healing may occur that resolve with no additional residual scarring, yet damages are claimed. Damages, depending on state law and jurisdictions, may include pain and suffering, loss of consortium, secondary and additional surgery, and delayed healing to name a few. It may be safe to assume that damages will be present should a breach of care occur. The more elective the surgery, the more careful the practice should be in accepting patients whose expectations and goals are reasonable and achievable.

Failure to meet expectations and financial considerations are the main reasons lawsuits are filed. It behooves a practice to spend an appropriate amount of time explaining, demonstrating, and providing visual aids to help patients make an informed decision about proceeding. I have always suggested that physicians, when possible, accept patients they "like" and in whom they will be able to provide a desired result. This may be difficult to achieve after only one visit. Prospective patients should be accepted only after they are seen at least twice, and surgical decisions are made.

Medicolegal Issues Inherent in Surgery of the Female Genitalia

Surgery in this anatomic area has many inherent risks and possible complications, which may occur even after the best care is provided. The general consent basically should include scarring, infection, bleeding, dyspareunia, nonhealing, the possible need for additional surgery and revisions, and less than desirable results. One trend of plaintiffs is to initiate a lawsuit because of an inherent risk such as a scar or a known complication. Surgeons should be careful beginning with the initial consult and throughout care to not imply, "This won't happen to you, but I have to talk about it." Evaluating and understanding additional patient risks that may interfere with care are essential. These include smoking, nutritional changes from dieting and weight-loss procedures, the effects from supplemental over-the-counter medications, and noncompliance with postoperative instructions and activity restrictions. Patients should be informed about the risks of noncompliance. Surgeons may say, "I can no longer be responsible for your outcome if you do not follow recommended instructions." All patients should sign a revision policy. The consent should clearly state the requirement to comply with preoperative and postoperative instructions and explain that noncompliant patients will be responsible for the cost of any additional surgery. For instance, labiaplasty patients who smoke before or after surgery are at a very high risk for wound complications. These patients should sign a revision policy stating that they will be required to pay for any revision surgery.

Surgeons who describe in advance a complication that occurs postoperatively are often thought to be very smart; however, the same information provided after the complication occurs is often seen as an excuse and is not well accepted. The best advice I can offer is to discuss the benefits of a procedure versus the inherent risks and complications that may occur, while ensuring the patient's goals are realistic. This process should be carried out over the course of several patient visits.

Informed consent is a critical component of a lawsuit and essential for patient happiness. Risk managers speak of informed consent, recognizing its importance, yet it is rarely the sole basis of a successful lawsuit. Cardiovascular studies suggested that patients understand and retain approximately 35% of what is discussed in a consultation.[1] However, these data are old, and by presenting information in a manner to accommodate patients' main learning styles—visual, auditory, and kinesthetic—rates of retention can be much higher. Through a collaborative effort of the surgeon, coordinator, nurse, and others, a practice can benefit by presenting a story of expectations for auditory learners, diagrams and photographs for visual learners, and specific examples of possible interactions for kinesthetic learners. The more all three are included in the informed consent process, the better a surgeon's understanding of the patient's expectations and the ability to achieve them, and the better the patient's understanding of acceptable risks and complications.

The informed consent process should be documented in an educational style and not in a legalese style. An appropriate amount of time should be allotted for questions and answers and to acknowledge that the patient understands what can, and especially what cannot, be achieved and that no results can be guaranteed. This cannot be accomplished in one visit, at the end of which the patient signs the reflection documentation, which is informed consent reflecting what has been discussed in this "process." Some patients never understand the informed consent process, whereas others do so after the second practice interaction. For those who do not understand, wise surgeons will not schedule surgery, but rather continue providing "nonselling" information, helping the prospective patient balance her goals and understanding. The process must be explained in part by the surgeon who will perform the surgery. The practice nurse or coordinator can assist but cannot thoroughly discuss and answer surgical questions.

Because of the varied anatomy of the genital area, new procedures, or more commonly variations of standard techniques, are necessary to achieve the best cosmetic results. Patients need to be informed of asymmetrical incisions such as those made for a unilateral double fold of the labia minora. A review of preoperative pictures (taken with the patient in a lithotomy position) is an important step with all cosmetic genital patients. The potential location of scars should be pointed out to patients before the surgery.

Before performing a new procedure or a variation of a standard technique, an experienced surgeon might say to a patient, "I am relying on my clinical experience and training." This is a reasonable statement, even though the procedure is one that is commonly performed. Often, such new procedures are variations of commonly performed, acceptable procedures that add a level of comfort for the surgeon and the patient. However, surgeons must disclose that this procedure is new. A suggested statement is: "This is a new and accepted procedure but certainly within my clinical training." The procedure should be based on sound, peer-reviewed, and accepted knowledge and articles. Arguably, a totally new procedure should have the patient safety of an Institutional Review Board. Variations of procedures using acceptable surgical technique may not require IRB involvement. This does not, however, obviate the need for a well-documented discussion of the procedure, experience related to it, risks, hazards, realistic goals, and alternatives. Failing to include such a discussion may lead to a patient, now a plaintiff, saying, "I never would have agreed to the procedure if I knew it was experimental and the doctor had no experience."

The patient's reasons and goals should be discussed. Failed expectations, a common reason for lawsuits, may arise when a patient does not thwart her husband's affair, rekindle romance, or achieve marital bliss. Through frank and open discussions during the informed consent process such desires may be revealed. Rarely does a surgical intervention adjust or correct marital or relationship problems. If a patient discloses that her reason for desiring surgery is to improve her marital sex relationship and overall intimacy and nothing is documented to dispel such a goal, an implied warranty may inadvertently be created. Once surgeons or team members hear information about an expectation that may not be achieved, they have a responsibility to state "that may not happen," and there are no warranties concerning the comment. Failing to dispel the stated expectation may create an implied warranty. Surgeons should be careful in advocating this new, exciting surgical field; appropriate patient selection with appropriate, achievable goals is essential.

Additional issues relating to informed consent include financial considerations. A clearly written, explicit financial agreement is needed that outlines costs, including the surgeon's fees, facility fees, anesthesia fees, lab pathology costs, and other expected and unexpected costs. A revision policy covering a finite period of time that the patient acknowledges in advance is advisable. I recommend that no additional surgical fees be included for necessary revisions within 1 year of surgery, provided that the patient complies with all scheduled follow-up instructions and visits. Additional fees for the facility and anesthesia may be necessary. This varies with each practice. What is important is that even if a surgeon waives revision costs, the patient may incur additional charges. Patients who do not follow instructions, miss appointments, smoke against medical advice, and create additional risks will not benefit from such a revision policy.

Surgeons can benefit from understanding warrantee issues. Two types of warranties may be established: express and implied. An *express warranty* is an exhibit, such as a photograph, drawing, or something demonstrative included in the record. It establishes what a patient thinks will be her expected result. When this result is not achieved, this express portion of the medical record possibly creates a breach of warranty. Therefore care is required in using visual aids to describe incisions, scars, and handling of issues to avoid implying that it is the expected result. When discussing photographs and schematics of results, surgeons should not imply that they show how all patients heal and results all patients achieve. Schematics showing a range of results and scarring should be discussed with patients to help them understand possible results, as opposed to implying results.

An *implied warranty* may be established if a patient discloses a specific goal or desire, and the surgeon knows that it may be difficult to achieve. For example, a patient discloses she has a very important business trip to a beach resort 2 weeks after surgery. Hearing this goal and not documenting a discussion with the patient of the difficulty of achieving it and the need to reschedule the surgery may establish an implied warranty that the patient will be able to attend this business meeting. Breach of warranty usually is not covered by general malpractice insurance, and it does not require negligence for a successful claim. The requirement is that a warranty is established and was not met. At least with a medical negligence claim, the defendant has an opportunity to prove that care was not negligent. A warranty should not be established, because only the warranty failure is needed to prove the claim.

Expectations and goals are critical in understanding a patient's desires and outside influences from partners and others. This surgery involves a large emotional component. A discussion with patients about their reasons for seeking such a surgery helps to determine their possible reaction if areas of nonhealing or additional scarring occurs. Surgeons should be very careful with patients who demand procedures or results that are either unrealistic or outside of an acceptable range. Accepting a patient, taking the patient's money, and operating on the patient for what may be a substandard result only because the patient wanted it is not acceptable. I have often stated that a patient cannot consent to a negligent procedure. A surgeon's responsibility and duty are to protect patients sometimes from themselves. Occasionally, a young labiaplasty patient will request a labiaplasty even though in a physical examination she has small labia minora. These patients should not undergo surgery, because the scarring and risks outweigh the potential cosmetic improvement. This may even result in not accepting patients regardless of how willing and demanding they are. We earn our living by patients we care for and our reputation by those we do not.

Surgeons must be mindful of having a chaperone always present during an examination. This even applies to female plastic surgeons and female patients. A patient's family member, female or otherwise, is not an acceptable chaperone. Should any abnormal or false complaint arise, it becomes their word against yours.

Privacy and communication issues have risen to a much higher concern in protecting patients' information data and confidentiality. Having a communication agreement that outlines how patients may be contacted, including via mail, email, home phone, work phone, cell phone, and/or social media, is essential. This consent for communication should be updated frequently and patient requests followed. If a patient's result is suitable to show to prospective patients, not only a HIPAA general consent is needed, but also a commercial HIPAA consent. This commercial consent should describe specifically where the photograph will be used, in what context, and for how long. It is absolutely necessary that the data embedded in the photograph be scrubbed, preventing any internal knowledge of the patient's identity. Ongoing privacy concerns should apply throughout the office, including all staff protecting the medical record, and even in public, should a patient be encountered in a social setting. I have told my patients that I will not be rude but will not acknowledge I know you to protect your privacy.

There are risks in every area of plastic surgery. Gorney and Martello[2] wrote significantly about balance between deformity and risks. His "Gorneygram" in Fig. 3-1 shows higher risks in treating patients with minimal deformities. Prospective patients with greater deformity and less concern (represented in the right lower side of the chart) tend to do much better than patients perceiving their minimal deformity as huge (represented in the upper left area of the chart). Caution is suggested when caring for patients whose balance of deformity and concern lies in this upper left area. This should be considered when counseling and treating patients seeking cosmetic improvement of the female genitalia. Although patients may have significant underlying emotional pressures, the proper procedure with improved results can be most satisfying.

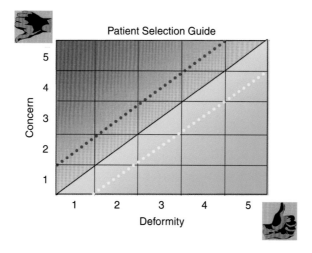

Fig. 3-1   The ratio of deformity on the horizontal axis to concern on the vertical axis helps to clarify patient expectations. A patient with a deformity level of 2 and a concern level of 4 may never be happy or find any result acceptable. Cautions apply! However, a patient with a deformity level of 4 and a concern level of 2 usually achieves an acceptable and rewarding result. Consider Quasimodo, the Hunchback of Notre Dame (deformity level of 5). He seeks hump improvement and states that any improvement will be great, because he understands that he will always have his hump (concern level of 2): This is an acceptable and realistic patient. However, a patient with a barely perceptible scar on her neck (deformity level of 1) but who refuses to leave her house without a turtleneck sweater to cover it (concern level of 5) may not be a realistic or acceptable patient. Patients whose profile is in the area between the *dotted lines* may be acceptable for care and treatment but only after very careful patient selection. For example, a patient whose profile is in the *red area* but between the dotted lines may be a candidate for surgery after many discussions.

Conclusion

This chapter is intended as a guideline and an aid in caring for patients considering or undergoing surgery of the female genitalia. Many more financial and psychological issues are involved. The team approach of a responsive and caring office can help patients most appropriately and provide a rewarding experience to all concerned.

References

1. Falagas ME, Korbila IP, Giannopoulou KP, et al. Informed consent: how much and what do patients understand? Am J Surg 198:420, 2009.
2. Gorney M, Martello J. Patient selection criteria. Clin Plast Surg 26:37, 1999.

Suggested Reading

American Society of Plastic Surgeons. Informed consent documents, edited by N. Reisman, 2012.

Part II
Techniques

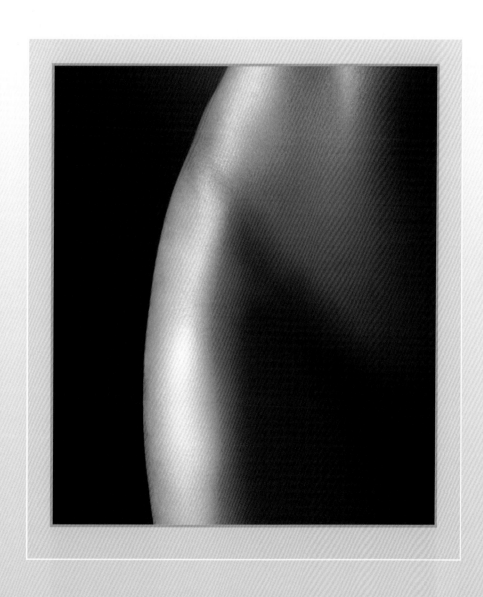

CHAPTER 4

Labial Reduction: Surgical Wedge Technique

Christine A. Hamori

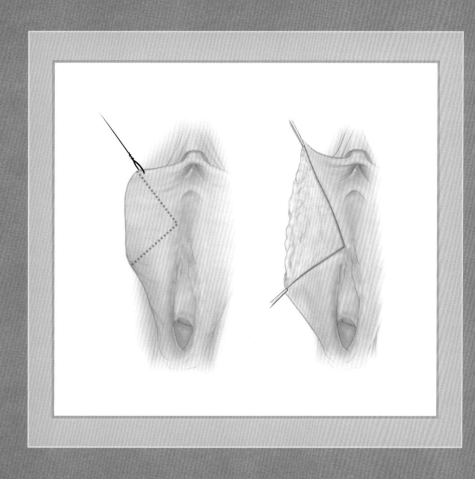

Key Points

- *Labiaplasty by wedge reduction is a safe and effective procedure.*

- *Wedge resection creates a small horizontal scar that is nearly imperceptible once healed.*

- *The removal of excess labia minora with a wedge technique spares critical nerves and preserves arterial supply.*

- *Patients tolerate the procedure well when given local anesthesia; it usually takes less than an hour to perform.*

- *The use of low-temperature plasma radiofrequency cautery may help in wound healing and early recovery.*

- *Complications such as edge notching, dehiscence, and hematoma are rare (see Chapter 10: Complications of Female Cosmetic Genital Surgery).*

Surgical alteration of the labia minora is the most frequently performed vaginal aesthetic procedure.[1] Many published techniques describe decreasing the size of the labia minora. The most common two types are edge trim procedures and wedge resections. In 1998 Alter[2] first described the wedge technique as a central wedge removed from the most protuberant portion of the labia minora. The advantages included preservation of the natural edge architecture, a shorter scar, and decreased scar sensitivity. In 2008 Alter[3] reviewed his 2-year experience with 407 extended wedge labiaplasties. The technical modification narrowed the clitoral hood and minimized the dog-ear created with the wedge-only technique. The incidence of complications was low, and the patient satisfaction rate was high.

Indications and Contraindications

Indications

Radial Elongation of the Labia Minora

Wedge techniques are best suited for patients with radial elongation of the labia and continuous edge pigmentation (Fig. 4-1). Basically, a simple "pie wedge" of full-thickness tissue is resected from the most protuberant portion of the labia minora, and the edges of the submucosa and mucosa are reapproximated. This pie wedge resection reduces the circumference thus reducing protrusion of the minora beyond the labia majora (Fig. 4-2).

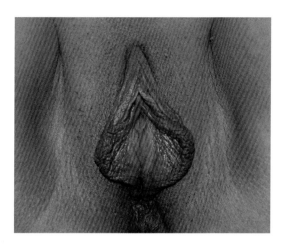

Fig. 4-1   This 49-year-old patient has a widened clitoral hood and labia minora excess.

A   B

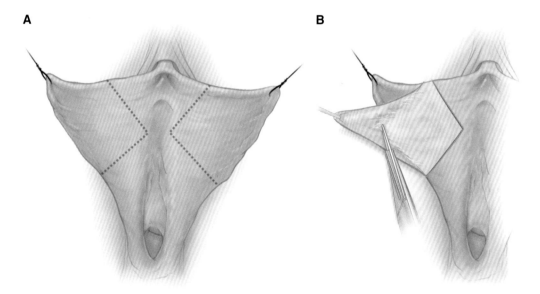

Fig. 4-2   A, Labia minora wedge resection markings. **B,** Excision of a wedge defect with preservation of the underlying submucosa.

Thickened Labia Minora

Thicker labia from mucosal or submucosal redundancy are suitable for wedge resections (Figs. 4-3 and 4-4). Edge trimming in such patents is difficult, because debulking submucosa necessitates near amputation of the labia. This results in labial remnants that are quite short and no longer have the natural edge architecture (Fig. 4-5). The wedge pro-

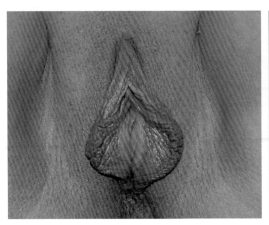 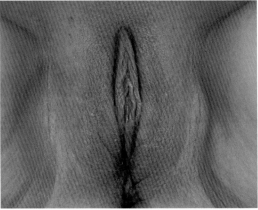

Fig. 4-3   This 49-year-old woman is shown before and 3 months after an extended wedge labiaplasty.

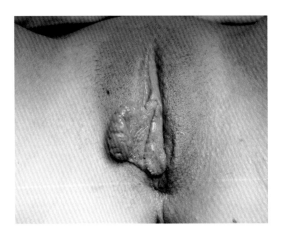

Fig. 4-4   This 27-year-old woman has unilateral labia minora hypertrophy (submucosal thickening).

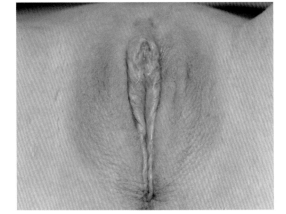

Fig. 4-5   This 46-year-old woman is shown 10 months after having an edge resection labiaplasty.

cedure allows adjustment of the amount of submucosa resection, facilitating the removal of full-thickness submucosa in patients with very bulky labia. However, in patients with thin or atrophic labia, the submucosa is preserved in the tissue remaining after a wedge resection (Figs. 4-6 and 4-7). Patients with minimal submucosa are also well suited for wedge resection.

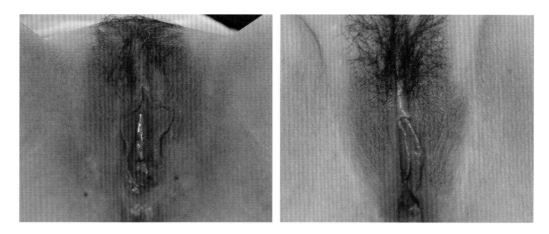

Fig. 4-6 This 44-year-old woman with thin, atrophic labia minora (minimal submucosa) is shown before and after an L-wedge resection by demucosalization.

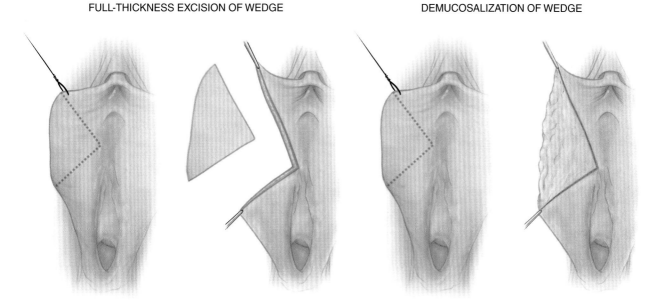

FULL-THICKNESS EXCISION OF WEDGE   DEMUCOSALIZATION OF WEDGE

Fig. 4-7 A full-thickness wedge resection for thick labia versus demucosalization for thin, atrophic labia.

Ruffled Variant

Patients with excess AP length in the sagittal plane or a ruffled variant are appropriate candidates for a series of small wedges along the length of the labia (Fig. 4-8). This reduces the length and thus the ruffling and bulkiness to provide a more aesthetic result (Fig. 4-9). A single, more obtuse wedge may suffice; however, tension would be greatest at the point of wedge closure, leaving curled and redundant tissue on either side of the

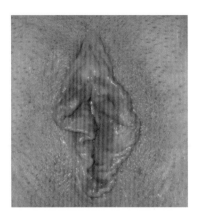

Fig. 4-8 This 40-year-old patient has ruffled labia minora excess in the sagittal plane.

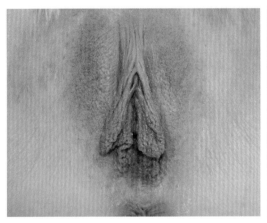
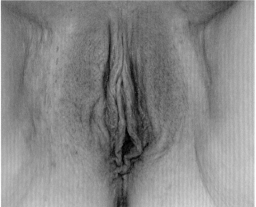

Fig. 4-9 This 37-year-old patient had redundant labia minora in the sagittal plane. She is shown before and after a wedge labiaplasty.

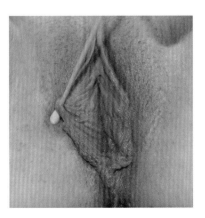

Fig. 4-10 This 32-year-old woman with thin labia minora has fenestrations 8 weeks after a wedge labiaplasty.

wedge. Very thin, atrophic labia with little submucosa are not amenable to wedge resection, because submucosal sutures tend to tear through, resulting in edge notching and/or fenestrations (Fig. 4-10).

Funnel Variant

Funnel-like labia minora that extend radially from a narrow base are a challenging anatomic variation (Fig. 4-11). These may be addressed with a conservative wedge resection or edge resection. In performing a wedge resection, noting the position of the posterior lip is essential. Aggressive wedge resection may result in impingement of the introitus posteriorly and discomfort during intercourse. The web should be released, similar to a small episiotomy, at the time of labiaplasty. This scar tends to be more painful postoperatively because of its location on the perineum. Using a hand mirror, surgeons should point out the posterior labial redundancy preoperatively and describe the additional scarring that will result.

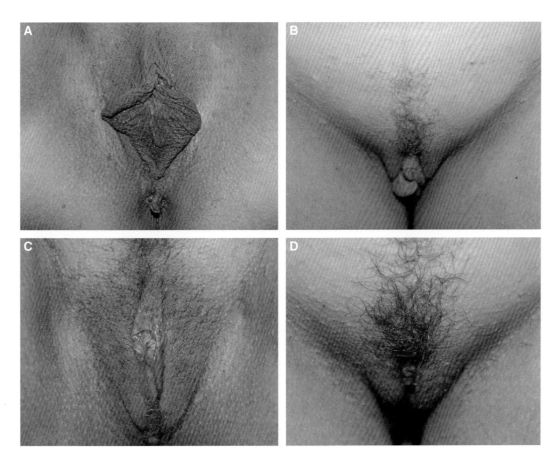

Fig. 4-11 A and **B,** This 46-year-old woman had a funnel variant. **C** and **D,** She is shown after having an extended wedge labiaplasty and posterior lip release.

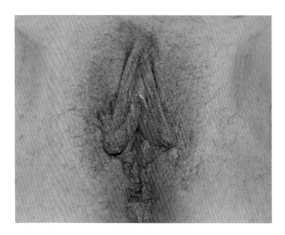

Fig. 4-12 This 50-year-old woman has a double-fold variant.

Double-Fold Variant

Many patients have additional folds of the labia minora superiorly. The fold begins at the confluence of the clitoral frenulum and the labia minora and extends superiorly for a variable distance toward the intervulvar commissure (Fig. 4-12). Patients with a unilateral double fold may not be aware of the fold preoperatively and should be shown the asymmetry during the consultation. Double folds are usually excised in a linear edge resection resulting in a scar in the interlabial groove. The scar tends to heal well, and excising the unilateral fold is typically recommended to prevent asymmetry postoperatively.

Widened Clitoral Hood

Patients with large labia minora may have a widened or redundant clitoral hood. Edge trim procedures in these patients may result in a persistence of hood laxity and redundancy and the appearance of a "penis" postoperatively[4] (Fig. 4-13). Hunter[5] stated that hood redundancy was the most common reason for revision labiaplasty surgery. The extended wedge procedure described by Alter[6] addresses the widened clitoral hood through a superior extension of the wedge onto the lateral clitoral hood (Fig. 4-14). The slight tension created by a wedge resection tends to reduce the anterior projection of the clitoral hood, preventing redundancy and the penis appearance.

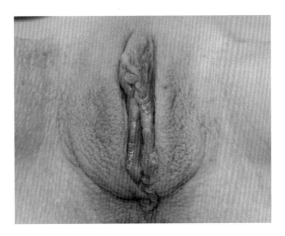

Fig. 4-13   This 41-year-old woman has a penis deformity after aggressive edge trim labiaplasty.

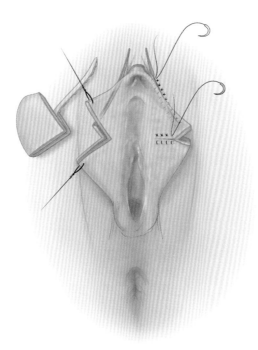

Fig. 4-14   Alter's extended wedge procedure[6] narrows the clitoral hood by a lateral extension.

Contraindications

The most common complication of wedge labiaplasty is edge dehiscence or notching. The incidence of wedge dehiscences and windows is much more common in smokers than in nonsmokers, probably because of the poor vascularization of the remaining labial flaps. Georgiou et al[7] showed that the labia minora are vascularized by branches of the internal and external pudendal arteries (Fig. 4-15). The dominant blood supply to the minora is through the internal pudendal vessel posteriorly. The large central artery, which courses perpendicular to the longest portion of the minora, supplies most of the labia minora. A small branch of the external pudendal system supplies the clitoral hood and the anterior-most portion of the labia minora. Wedge resections placed posteriorly (posterior wedge resection) over the central artery may induce ischemia of the anterior labial wedge flap, which is supplied only by small vessels from the external pudendal system. For patients with compromised vascularity, such as smokers, surgeons should consider an edge trim resection instead of a wedge resection. According to the authors, edge trim labiaplasty maintained consistent flap vascularity along the labial edge (Fig. 4-16).

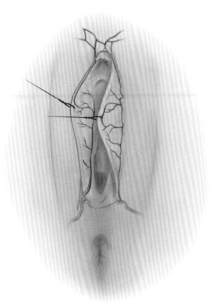

Fig. 4-15 Arterial anatomy of the labia minora with dominant superior circulation.

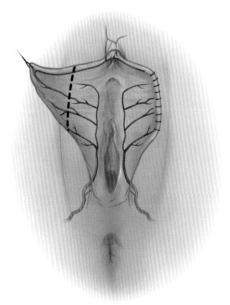

Fig. 4-16 The result after labia minora trimming. No arterial compromise of the remaining labia minora is evident.

Inadequate length of the minora in the anteroposterior direction is a contraindication to wedge labiaplasty. Wedge resection in such anatomic variants may result in excess tension on the closure, with resulting wound separation. In patients with pigmentation variation along the minora, the dark labia must not be opposed with lighter labia, which would cause a stripe. In these patients, an edge trim may help to remove the pigmented edge for a more aesthetic result.

Patient Evaluation

In assessing patients for labial surgery, understanding their goals and expectations is critical. A brief sexual and gynecologic history should be obtained. Once a patient describes her desires she is shown the basic anatomy, and surgical options, risks, and potential complications are discussed. The external genitalia are examined. Having another medical person in the room during the pelvic examination is advised. The labia minora are assessed for redundancy, asymmetry, and pigmentation. The labia majora and clitoral hood are examined.

The patient is given a mirror and asked to indicate areas that are particularly bothersome. The surgeon identifies the proposed incision location. It is important to emphasize that asymmetry is very common in this area, and that a certain amount of asymmetry will remain postoperatively. Combined procedures such as clitoral hood reduction and labia majora reduction may be discussed during the examination phase of the consultation.

Preoperative Planning and Preparation

At the consultation, the surgeon and patient discuss the proposed surgery and the potential risks and complications. Diagram templates in the electronic record are useful for sketching the proposed procedure during the consultation.

Because of the delicate and potentially embarrassing nature of the surgery, photographs are not taken until the morning of the day of surgery. If the procedure will be done with the patient under a local anesthetic, an oral cephalosporin antibiotic is given 30 minutes preoperatively. Anterior and posterior photographs are obtained while the patient is standing with her legs spread slightly in front of a solid background (Fig. 4-17, *A*). This helps to document the amount of protrusion beyond the majora, the size and position of the labia majora, and asymmetries. When the patient is in the operating room and in stirrups, photographs are taken while she is in a lithotomy position (Fig. 4-17, *B*).

Labiaplasty may be performed with the patient under local or general anesthesia. Patients younger than 25 years of age and those who are anxious and have difficulty being examined while in the lithotomy position at the consultation are sedated intravenously or

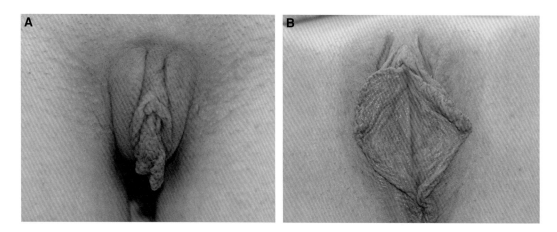

Fig. 4-17   Preoperative **A,** standing and **B,** lithotomy photos of a 28-year-old woman with labia minora and clitoral hood enlargement.

given general anesthesia. These patients do not need topical anesthetics and are given an intravenous antibiotic (a first-generation cephalosporin) 30 minutes before the procedure. Lidocaine with epinephrine, as described later, is injected for hemostasis.

Local anesthesia alone or in combination with oral sedation such as Percocet and Valium works well for most patients. Topical application of benzocaine, lidocaine, and tetracaine 20 minutes before the procedure is effective. Patients usually do not feel the injections if they are given very slowly with a 30-gauge needle, starting on the mucosal side of the minora. The mucosa is more easily distended with lidocaine, resulting in minimal if any pain. Injections in the interlabial crease, between the lateral minora and the labia majora, are needed for an extended wedge technique and may be uncomfortable, because the skin is thicker in this area.

Surgical Technique

Markings

Markings are made after the photographs of the patient in the lithotomy position have been taken. The labial wedge is marked as anteriorly as possible. The anterior limb is drawn first, and the labium is folded to approximate the more posterior limb of the V. The more anterior limb must not be placed too close (less than 0.5 cm) to the urethral meatus, because distortion may result in spraying of the urinary stream. The two edges of the V should approximate with minimal if any tension. Once one side is completed, the other labium is marked. The two marked wedges may be of different size based on the redundancy of the labia minora. If the patient has a connected posterior fourchette that is pulled anteriorly with approximation of the wedge resections, the fourchette is released. A single incision centrally on the web of the fourchette is drawn in the sagittal plane.

Coaptation of the edges of the labial defect with minimal tension is imperative. The markings are performed before local anesthesia is injected. The wedge is centralized around the most prominent portion of the labia minora and maintained as anteriorly as possible to maximize adequate blood supply[7] (Figs. 4-18 and 4-19). In marking the anteriormost portion of the wedge, the confluence of the clitoral frenulum, the clitoral hood, and the labia minora must be considered. An incision above the confluence will result in a W-shaped flap that will need to be anastomosed to the single-edged posterior flap.

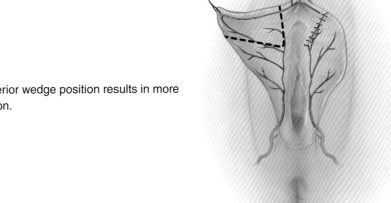

Fig. 4-18 An anterior wedge position results in more robust flap perfusion.

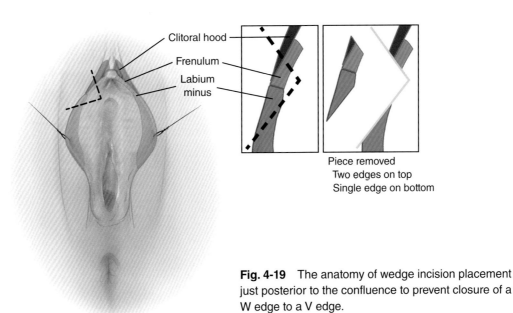

Clitoral hood
Frenulum
Labium minus

Piece removed
Two edges on top
Single edge on bottom

Fig. 4-19 The anatomy of wedge incision placement just posterior to the confluence to prevent closure of a W edge to a V edge.

Anesthesia

Once the markings are completed, 1% lidocaine with epinephrine 1:100,000 is injected (using a 30-gauge needle) submucosally along the wedge markings and superiorly in the interlabial groove. At least 10 minutes is needed for the anesthetic and epinephrine to take effect. If the procedure is performed with the patient under local anesthesia, a topical anesthetic (benzocaine 20%, lidocaine 6%, tetracaine 4%) is applied to the area and requires 15 minutes to take effect. One dose of a second-generation cephalosporin antibiotic is given preoperatively either orally or intravenously, depending on the type of anesthesia given.

Patient Positioning

The patient is brought into the operating room and placed in a lithotomy position with the legs secured in boot-type stirrups to provide calf and foot support. Photographs are taken (Fig. 4-20). The labia minora are photographed while they are abducted and ad-

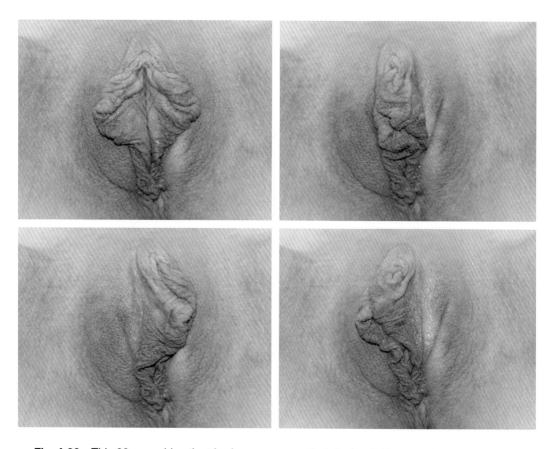

Fig. 4-20 This 28-year-old patient is shown preoperatively before labiaplasty (lithotomy views).

ducted to document asymmetries in length, the presence of a unilateral or bilateral double fold, the presence of a posterior confluence of the minora, and clitoral hood variations. These variations merit special attention intraoperatively to achieve symmetry and prevent surgical revisions.

Technique

The incisions are made through the mucosa with a No. 15 blade, a Peak PlasmaBlade (Medtronic), or a needle-point cautery device. The lower temperature (40° to 100° C) of the plasma device versus the temperature of traditional electrocautery has been shown to decrease thermal injury and improve wound healing in surgical wounds.[8,9] Submucosal resection is conservative in most patients. In patients with very atrophic, thin labia minora, it is best to demucosalize the wedge rather than perform a full-thickness resection. Hemostasis is obtained with cautery, and Marcaine 0.05% with 1:200,000 epinephrine is injected in the area.

Once hemostasis is confirmed, the wedge defect is closed from deep to superficial with monofilament absorbable suture such as 4-0 Monocryl on an SH taper needle. Buried sutures are placed between the dermis of the anterior wedge and the posterior wedge. Approximately five of these sutures are needed per labia. The leading edge is meticulously reapproximated with a vertical mattress suture of 5-0 Monocryl on an RU taper needle. This suture helps to prevent notching. If a dog-ear forms laterally after the wedge closure or if the clitoral hood is wide, a narrow triangle of superolateral labia minora may be resected, placing the scar along the interlabial groove. The final mucosal layer is closed with interrupted or running absorbable suture of 5-0 Vicryl Rapide or 5-0 Monocryl.

Postoperative Care

The incisions are cleaned with a sodium solution, and a topical antibiotic ointment is applied. A disposable Perineal Cold Pack and pad (Medline Industries) are applied, and a webbed, disposable mesh panty is placed. Marcaine provides approximately 4 hours of analgesia, after which patients may have pain manifested as burning. They are instructed to take Vicodin every 4 to 6 hours as necessary for the next 24 to 48 hours. At discharge patients are given a perineal irrigation bottle and instructions to spray warm water over the incisions after micturition. For patients older than 35 years of age, a topical conjugated estrogen (Premarin) is prescribed with instructions to apply the medication to the area three times per week for 6 weeks. This promotes wound healing. An oral, second-generation antibiotic (Duricef) is prescribed with instructions to take it twice daily for 5 days. Patients with itching and discharge are given an oral antifungal such as Diflucan.

Results and Outcomes

Extended Wedge Labiaplasty With Posterior Fourchette Release

This 32-year-old female had excess labia minora. She was so embarrassed by the appearance that she avoided having sex. She wanted as little labial show as possible. On her standing examination, she had a widened intervulvar commissure with dangling labia minora. In a lithotomy position, her minora were redundant with thickening of the leading edge. She had a connected posterior fourchette and a gradation of pigmentation from light anteriorly to dark posteriorly (Fig. 4-21, *A* and *B*).

An extended wedge labiaplasty with a posterior fourchette release was performed. The patient tolerated the procedure well. Postoperatively, she has less separation of the intervulvar commissure because of the reduced labia minora and narrowed clitoral hood. She has a slight difference in pigmentation at the site of the wedge incision (Fig. 4-21, *B* and *C*).

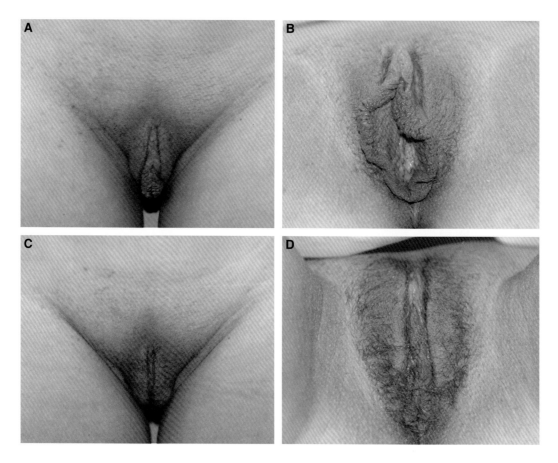

Fig. 4-21   A and **B,** This 32-year-old patient is shown before having an extended wedge labiaplasty with a posterior fourchette release. **C** and **D,** Postoperative result.

Extended Wedge Labiaplasty With an Inverted-V Clitoral Hood Reduction

This 55-year-old female had redundant, pointy labia minora and elongation of the clitoral hood. The labia minora tended to protrude from beneath her underwear. While she was standing, the labia minora appeared long, the intervulvar commissure was narrow, and the clitoral hood was slightly elongated but narrow. In a lithotomy position, she had narrow-based, elongated labia minora with some pigmentation and thickened submucosa. The clitoral hood was narrow but long, extended beyond the clitoris, and appeared atrophic. The clitoris was not enlarged (Fig. 4-22, *A* and *B*).

An extended wedge labiaplasty was performed with an inverted-V clitoral hood reduction. Postoperatively, the patient did well and was happy with the result. Her postoperative lithotomy photo shows shortening of the clitoral hood with no perceptible scar across the dorsum of the hood. The labia minora are smaller and thinner. In the standing photo, the minora do not dangle beyond the majora (Fig. 4-22, *C* and *D*).

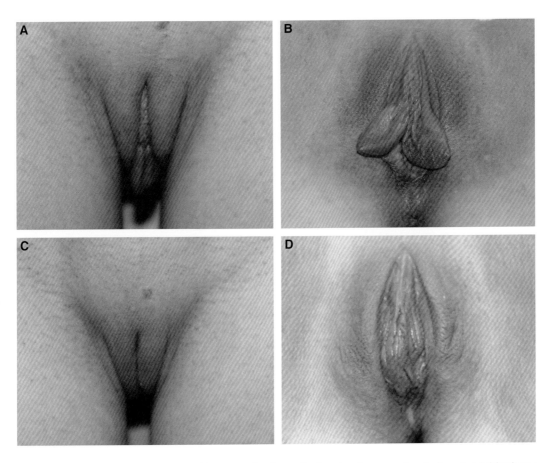

Fig. 4-22 A and **B,** This 55-year-old woman is shown before having an extended wedge labiaplasty and a clitoral hood reduction. **C** and **D,** Postoperative result.

Problems and Complications

Postoperative complications from wedge labiaplasty include wound dehiscence, hematoma, pigment mismatch, and inadequate labial reduction. Wound dehiscence by far is the most common problem postoperatively, especially in smokers (see Fig. 10-2). This can be prevented by minimizing the size of the wedge to decrease tension and by placing the wedge as anteriorly as possible to prevent transection of the dominant central artery. In smokers, edge trims are recommended, avoiding wedge resection altogether.

Hematomas that form postoperatively usually occur within the first 24 to 48 hours. Small hematomas present with asymmetrical swelling and pain. Patients should be evaluated, but surgical intervention is rarely necessary. Larger hematomas require surgical evacuation in the operating room usually with patients under general anesthesia.

The demand for female aesthetic surgery continues to rise rapidly. Further studies are needed to investigate long-term outcomes.[10] An extended wedge labiaplasty is a simple and effective technique to reduce the size and protrusion of the labia minora. It is best employed in patients with thicker labia minora (excess submucosa) and in those with clitoral hood redundancy in the sagittal plane. Attention to hemostasis and edge alignment is essential to prevent complications such as notching, edge dehiscence, and hematomas. Complications from wedge labiaplasty are discussed in Chapter 10.

References

1. Goodman MD, Michael P, Placik OJ, et al. A large multicenter outcome study of female genital plastic surgery. J Sex Med 7:1565, 2010.
2. Alter GJ. A new technique for aesthetic labia minora reduction. Ann Plast Surg 40:287, 1998.
3. Alter GJ. Aesthetic labia minora and clitoral hood reduction using extended central wedge resection. Plast Reconstr Surg 122:1780, 2008.
4. Hamori CA. Postoperative clitoral hood deformity after labiaplasty. Aesthet Surg J 33:1030, 2013.
5. Hunter JG. Labia minora, labia majora, and clitoral hood alteration: experience-based recommendations. Aesthet Surg J 36:71, 2016.
6. Alter GJ. Central wedge (Alter) labia minora reduction. Int Soc Sex Med 12:1514, 2015.
7. Georgiou CA, Benatar M, Dumas P, et al. A cadaveric study of the arterial blood supply of the labia minora. Plast Reconstr Surg 136:167, 2015.
8. Ruidaz ME, Messmer D, Atmodjo DY, et al. Comparative healing of human cutaneous surgical incisions created by the PEAK PlasmaBlade, conventional electrosurgery, and a standard scalpel. Plast Reconstr Surg 128:104, 2011.
9. Isik F. Discussion: comparative healing of human cutaneous surgical incisions created by the PEAK PlasmaBlade, conventional electrosurgery, and a standard scalpel. Plast Reconstr Surg 128:112, 2011.
10. Lista F, Mistry BD, Singh Y, et al. The safety of aesthetic labiaplasty: a plastic surgery experience. Aesthet Surg J 35:689, 2015.

CHAPTER 5

Labia Minora Reduction Surgery: Curved Linear Resection

Red Alinsod

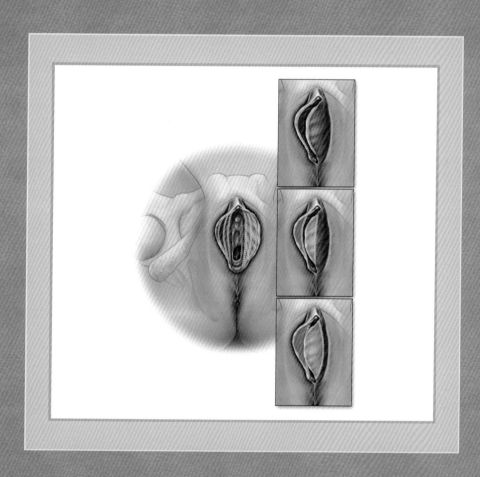

Key Points

- Most gynecologists who perform labiaplasty surgery use curved linear resection. In a survey of plastic surgeons who performed labia minoraplasties, the most commonly performed technique was curved linear resection (52.7%) followed by central V wedge resection (36.1%).[1]

- Although the edge excision technique reportedly has fewer wound-healing complications, it leaves a suture line at the periphery that may rarely result in scar contracture and rare chronic pain during coitus.[2] Wedge excisions leave the same type of scar but in a mostly horizontal manner. Scars causing pain are exceptionally rare, because labial scars dramatically diminish and soften and are generally not detectable within 6 months for both wedge excisions and linear excisions.

- Different techniques may be preferable for different patients, depending on the advantages and disadvantages of the procedure, the degree and location of labia minora hypertrophy, and the patient's cosmetic preference. Generally, curved linear excision provides patients with any degree of cosmetic appearance they desire but does not maintain the appearance of the dark and irregular edges. The more radical reductions are not possible with wedge techniques.

- Most women undergoing minoraplasty want the dark edges of the labia minora removed, but some prefer to preserve the dark natural-looking edge and request only reduction of the labial bulk.[2,3] More aggressive resections and exacting excisions are possible with curved linear resections as opposed to wedge techniques.

- Emerging evidence supports the increased safety, precision, functional, and aesthetics of radiofrequency (RF) labia minora labiaplasty, compared with other minora reduction procedures, performed by a properly trained and experienced practitioner.[4]

Labiaplasty, which is sometimes called *labioplasty,* is a gynecologic surgical procedure to reduce the size and sometimes the shape of either the labia majora or labia minora.[5,6] It is currently one of the most frequently performed aesthetic vaginal surgical procedures.[5] The bilateral longitudinal mucocutaneous folds between the labia majora and vulvar vestibule are called *nymphae* or *labia minora.*[6-8] The labia minora are extremely sensitive to touch during sexual stimulation because of the erectile connective tissue and rich nerve endings in the nymphae.[5] The minora vary widely in length, thickness, symmetry, protuberance, and the degree to which they project beyond the edge of the labia majora.[5,6,8,9] Rarely, the minora protrude more than 3 cm beyond the free edge of the labia majora[5-10] and are often considered hypertrophic and aesthetically displeasing. The cause of hypertrophic labia minora can be multifactorial and includes congenital[8,11] and acquired idiopathic hypertrophy[12,13] from intercourse or possibly masturbation, childbirth by the vaginal route, lymphatic stasis, inflammation from dermatitis or urinary incontinence,[5] and stretching with weights and exogenous androgenic hormones.[13]

In 1984 Hodgkinson and Hait[14] described their experiences with labiaplasty on three women unhappy with the size and bulkiness of their labia minora. Their study led to the first published report on elective cosmetic reduction surgery of the labia minora designed for visual improvement of the external genitalia in Western women. The main surgical techniques currently used in labia minora reduction include curved linear excision (sometimes referred to as *cutting* or *amputation* techniques) or elliptical excision[3,8,14] (also called *longitudinal resection* or *trimming* of the labial edges with oversewing of the labial edge),[3,15,16] central wedge resection,[17] modified V-wedge resection (V plasty),[18,19] deepithelialization,[13,20] laser labiaplasty,[21] and RF labiaplasty. Regardless of the technique employed, labia minoraplasty procedures should not damage the neurovascular supply or the introitus. A viable labiaplasty should preserve the contour of the lips, when requested by the patient, and the color and texture of the labial edge, or the labia minora should be removed , if requested.[3,8] Patients are given an in-office, local anesthetic (0.25% Marcaine or 1% lidocaine with 1:100,000 epinephrine), conscious sedation, or traditional general anesthesia.[3,5]

In 2005 I reported on a minimally invasive surgical procedure popularly called the *Barbie look* (Fig. 5-1).[3] This is a slang term used by patients in Los Angeles who requested removal of all or almost all of the labia minora. The *rim look* and the *hybrid look* procedures were

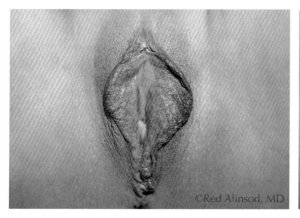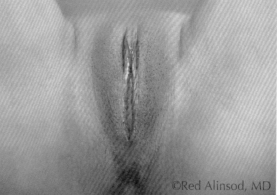

Fig. 5-1 This patient is shown before and after having a Barbie look procedure.

also described (Figs. 5-2 and 5-3). The rim look procedure involves a curved linear vertical excision of only the dark edges of the labia minora to smoothen and even them. They should protrude past the labia majora. The hybrid look refers to a finessed, middle-road approach involving removal of nearly all of the labia minora and preservation of a petite "peekaboo" (below or to the level of the labia majora) amount of tissue that appears more attractive to some patients.[3] This degree of precise excision of labial tissue is possible with the use of RF pinpoint "hair" tips. This exact degree of tissue removal cannot be satisfactorily achieved with wedge techniques.

Regional preferences for the Barbie look vary significantly, with a greater preference reported on the West Coast than on the East Coast or in the South. In a study of 238 women considering labial reduction, 98% sought a labia minora reduction to the level of or below the level of the labia majora.[22] In my survey[4] of 200 patients, none preferred

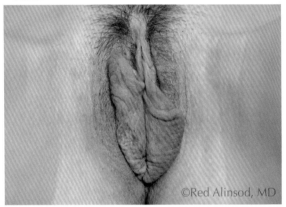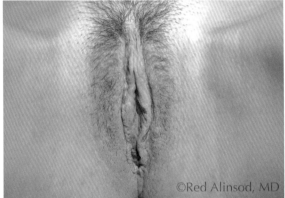

Fig. 5-2   This patient is shown before and after having a rim labiaplasty.

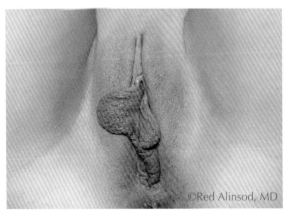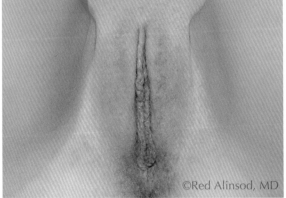

Fig. 5-3   This patient is shown before and after having a hybrid labiaplasty.

to retain the contour and/or darkness of the corrugated free edge. Instead, all patients requested removal rather than retention of the dark edges. In my experience, it is extremely rare for a woman to ask her surgeon to leave the dark labial edges intact during a labiaplasty. In Miklos and Moore's study[22] of 550 women, 97% wanted removal of the dark edges (preferring pink edges), which resulted in a smoother contour of the labial free edge.

Wedge techniques are ideal for females seeking to retain the dark edges or the natural contours of the labia minora. A wedge resection, a full-thickness excision, and modifications of this technique are sometimes preferable for minimizing nerve injury, scarring, and overresection that can lead to an excessively tightened introitus.[8,11] In 1998 Alter[11] introduced modifications of the wedge resection, including a central wedge resection with an external wedge (hockey stick V),[8,17] a 90-degree Z-plasty,[5,7] an inferior wedge resection,[23] and Maas and Hage's zigzag technique.[8,24]

An extended central wedge resection incorporates an external wedge (hockey stick V) to remove excess lateral clitoral hooding or dog-ears.[8,17] This approach is associated with less wound edge separation, sinus/fistula formation, clitoral hood excess, and postoperative pain, although absolute numbers of affected patients are limited and the number of patients with these complications is not always reported.[8] The addition of a 90-degree Z-plasty to the central wedge excision spreads the tension over the suture line, thus minimizing traction on the suture line.[5,7] In an inferior wedge resection approach, the wedge is removed in the inferior part of the labia, and the superior pedicle is used to reconstruct the labia.[23] Maas and Hage's zigzag technique[8,24] is another modification of a wedge excision. It involves a W-shaped resection with interdigitated suturing of the protuberant labium. The downsides of wedge-type labiaplasty surgery are the variable blood supply of the labia and the tension on the outward pulling edges. Wedge-type labiaplasty carries increased risk for improper healing, holes in the labia, and distinct pizza-shaped gaps when the edges pull apart.[3] These complications have not been reported in curved linear resections performed by qualified surgeons. Surgical techniques may be combined, if warranted, with different methods sometimes used on each labium.[8]

In bilateral deepithelialization both the medial and lateral sides of each small vaginal lip are marked to delineate excisable areas, and both sides are deepithelialized, or "skinned off," with either a scalpel or laser. The procedure is performed in approximately 30 minutes. The technique is advantageous if only a minimal amount of labia tissue needs to be excised.[25] However, if a large area must be deepithelialized, the approach may result in a redundant free border, increased labial thickness with bunching, wound necrosis and breakdown, and an abrupt color change at the suture line.[5,25] Laser labiaplasty has not been shown to be advantageous in repairing the labial edge after the excess tissue is trimmed. Although laser labiaplasty is used in the deepithelialization technique, it increases the risk for development of epidermal inclusion cysts.[5] Furthermore, deepithelialization can interfere with the labial blood supply, resulting in holes and gaps in healing.[4]

Alinsod Surgical Technique for Radiofrequency Labia Minoraplasty

In the past decade the use of RF-based excision and revision surgery in aesthetic vulvovaginal surgery has increased. RF labiaplasty was first performed and reported in 2005 and presented in 2006[3] at the meeting for the American Academy of Cosmetic Gynecologists. This technique is especially suitable for labiaplasty surgery, because the minimal lateral thermal spread is only 20 to 40 μm when the procedure is performed with a hair-tip attachment. No discernable edge burn or scarring is visible, and no bubbling of skin occurs. Both of these features lead to improved safety during delicate surgery around the clitoral region. RF technology also allows feathering of irregular edges and smoothening and flattening of the dog-ears.

RF incisional and excisional surgery can be performed with all techniques described. It is most frequently used with curved linear excisions. This technique is described at length here.

Indications and Contraindications

Labia minora reduction surgery may be performed for functional or aesthetic reasons or both. Functional indications of labia minoraplasty include difficulty maintaining hygiene (for example, because toilet paper sticks), chronic chafing of the pudendal skin, irritation when wearing tight clothing, pain during bicycle riding and similar sports activities, and the labia catching in zippers.[5,9,15,18,25] Many women undergo labiaplasty for aesthetic reasons, particularly because of the appearance of a bulge under their clothing [3,5,19,25] or because of enlarged inner vaginal lips that cause embarrassment during sexual relations.[18,26] Because the causes for undergoing this procedure typically involve both cosmetic and functional issues, labia minoraplasty is equally a medical therapeutic intervention and a cosmetic surgical procedure. There are no absolute contraindications to labiaplasty; relative contraindications include active gynecologic infections and malignancy.[5]

Patient Evaluation

Patient consultations are preferably carried out days before surgery but may occur on the same day as surgery, with special arrangements such as a prior Internet consultation. For example, an athletic runner may present in the office with complaints of uneven labia that are embarrassing and painful. Her prior rectocele repair was successful but resulted in asymmetrical labia, with a constant pulling sensation. She requests a labiaplasty to remove almost all the labia minora on both sides, preserving a small amount of labia for a more natural look. The patient is given a mirror to ensure that she and the surgeon are discussing the same structures. On physical examination, the left labia are twice the size of the right labia and are thicker with darker edges. She may request a more symmetrical appearance and removal of the darkened edges. The clitoral hood is not bothersome to the patient, but she does not want a "top heavy" look after labial reduction. A clitoral hood reduction is recommended for some patients to provide a more symmetrical appearance. Preoperative photographs are taken with the patient in various positions. Examining the patient when she is lying down and standing can help to show the anatomy involved and to confirm the requested amount of labial tissue to remove and the desired, ideal appearance. They are reviewed with the patient so that she can envision the appearance of her labia once they are healed and to help her decide the amount of labia to remove and whether a clitoral hood reduction would be aesthetically beneficial.

Preoperative Planning and Preparation

After extensive discussions with the patient, a decision is made and documented with drawings and/or photographs. The patient is screened for her general health, allergies, pregnancy status, anxiety, tolerance to pain, understanding of the procedure, and a detailed consent is obtained.

Anesthesia

Approximately 2 hours before surgery, the patient places numbing cream (EMLA or compounded topical anesthetics) on the surgical sites. When labiaplasty is carried out in the office, dermoelectroporation is performed for 15 to 30 minutes to push the macromolecular numbing cream under the skin to provide comfort during the placement of local anesthesia (Fig. 5-4). Oral or intramuscular narcotics are given in combination with an anxiolytic agent such as Valium.

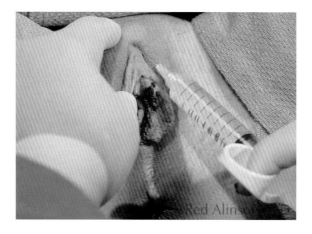

Fig. 5-4 A local anesthetic is injected.

Markings

Markings are made with a surgical marker starting laterally and below the frenulum and extending down to the introitus (Fig. 5-5). Because more lateral tissue retraction always occurs on the upper third of the labia minora, markings are adjusted by a slow tapering down of approximately 1.5 cm below the frenulum, to a nearly total absence of labia at the introitus. The medial side of the minora is similarly marked, and markings to delineate the matched shape and size are made on the opposite labia. The patient's requested amount of labia minora to protrude past the labia majora is considered, and markings are adjusted accordingly. Conservative placement of markings is recommended, because it is better to leave more labia than to remove too much. Removal of slightly more medial minora while leaving a slightly wider lateral minora will result in a medially hidden surgical scar.

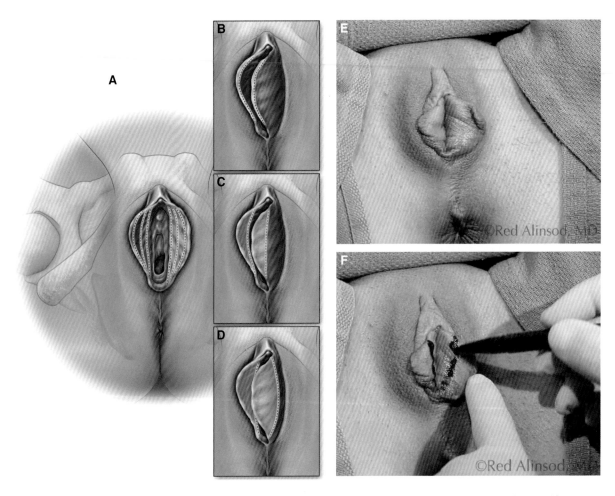

Fig. 5-5   A, Markings for a deepithelialization technique. **B,** Removal of only the labial edge (rim look). **C,** Removal of most of the labia at or below the level of the labia majora (hybrid look). **D,** Removal of all or almost all of the labia minora (Barbie look). **E,** The patient is shown preoperatively. **F,** Markings are made.

Patient Positioning

The patient is placed in a low lithotomy position, with adequate support of the legs to ensure comfort and good blood flow. Support under the knees and calf is recommended over simple heel support.

Technique

The vulvar region is prepped in the standard manner with Betadine or an equivalent. Sterile towels or a drape system is placed, and the patient is made comfortable. Re-marking is typically needed after a prep that may fade the initial markings. Approximately 4 to 7 ml of the anesthetic is injected just under the skin, subcuticularly, in all marked areas. A very small-gauge needle is recommended. This microtumescent technique prevents tissue distortion. The area is checked for adequate anesthesia to confirm numbness of all surgical incision sites.

The incision is started 1 to 1.5 cm below the frenulum and over the markings and extended down to the introitus or perineum, depending on the precise location on the bottom to which the labia minora is attached (Fig. 5-6, *A* and *B*). At the time of this writing, in the United States only, the Surgitron and Pellevé systems (Ellman International, Hicksville, NY) have handpieces that can accommodate a fine, pinpoint hair tip for excisional labiaplasty. The Cutting mode at 10 to 15 watts is used for excision, and the Blend or Coag mode at 20 to 25 watts is used for hemostasis. A third mode, the Hemo mode, at higher wattage, can help to control bleeding and is useful for "brushing" irregularities to make them flat and smooth. Tissue can be substantially debulked by making angled incisions toward the middle of the labia minora from the medial and lateral sides. This technique leaves a small "canal" that causes the edges of the minora to cling together as they fall medially toward it. Standard cautery and 980-diode lasers are not effective because of

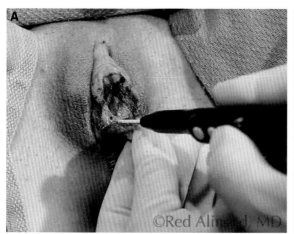 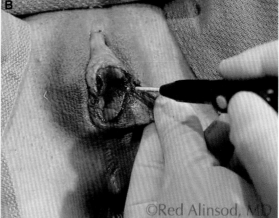

Fig. 5-6   A and **B,** An RF excision is performed.

their coagulation-inducing properties that may cause distortion and inward crimping of the labial edges. Once hemostasis is obtained, refinements can be made (Fig. 5-6, *C*). "A" incisions, also referred to as *Alinsod incisions* are made below or lateral to the frenulum to hide the suture line medially (Fig. 5-6, *D* and *E*). This helps remove potential "dog-ears" and helps hide suture lines. This is the most difficult part of the procedure and one that demands strategic forward thinking to achieve beautiful results. Enhanced symmetry, improved alignment, and matching of the edges can be accomplished using the ultrafine hair tip at strategic locations. This stage is the optimal time to show the patient the progress made in the surgery and the degree of labial tissue excised. The patient can visualize the surgical site with a handheld mirror and help to guide the clinician's remaining surgical tasks, if needed, by either approving the outcome or requesting further refinements.

In our practice the procedure is done with the patient awake so that she can approve the degree of tissue reduction shown to her by a mirror. A layered closure is initiated (Fig. 5-6, *F*). Absorbable 4-0 or 5-5 monofilament, such as Monocryl, is best for the deepest

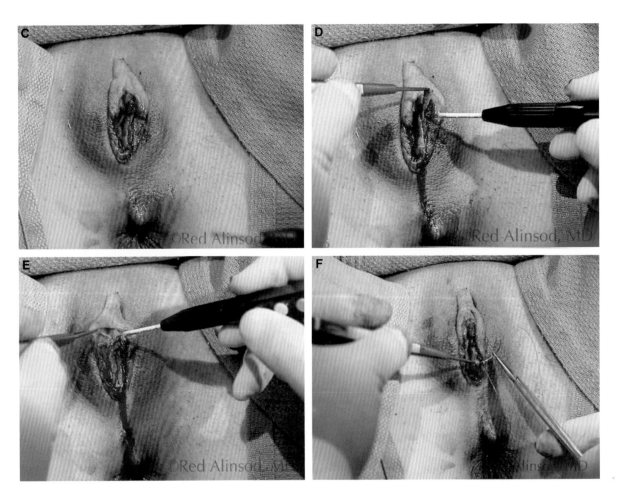

Fig. 5-6, cont'd   C, The clitoral hood is evaluated. **D** and **E,** An A incision is made. **F,** Layered suturing is performed.

suturing. It resists premature suture breakdown often seen with multifilament materials such as synthetic absorbable sutures primarily composed of polyglycolic acid, including polyglactin 910 (for example, Vicryl), and other polyglycolic acid sutures treated for accelerated breakdown (for example, Vicryl Rapide). Vicryl is ideal as the last layer of interrupted refinement sutures, because they do not poke the surrounding tissues. There is no role for catgut sutures in these surgeries, because they increase the risk for local hypersensitivity reactions to materials derived from chromic gut. Suturing is done with fine needles such as a tapered SH. Smaller needles are effective, but surgeons should not use cutting needles, which may cause additional tissue damage.

The principles of labial closure should be defined. First, the deeper dead spaces with larger vessels must be closed gently to prevent abscess or hematoma formation. Loose but secure suturing will reduce clumping of tissues and rigid edge scarring. No entrapped skin should remain, because it can cause inclusion cysts to form. The deeper stitches can be interrupted, but inverted mattress sutures will better align the edges during side-to-side stitching. Second, a layer of subcuticular sutures of 4-0 or 5-0 Vicryl or Monocryl will hold lined up edges together. Last, several strategically placed 4-0 sutures should be placed loosely along the full length of the labial edges bilaterally. The patient is asked to view the final results and to give her feedback and suggestions. If she is satisfied, the remaining local anesthetic can be injected to prolong the anesthetic effects.

Postoperative Care

Routine postoperative care instructions are reviewed. No exercise or heavy lifting or sexual activity is instructed for the next 6 weeks, although gentle and slow-paced walking is allowed. The surgical site should be cleaned daily with soap and water and pat dried without rubbing. There is no soaking in tubs of water and no Sitz baths allowed. That may weaken sutures and result in premature wound opening. The patient is instructed to place estradiol cream on the labia and over the wound sites daily to aid healing. Collagen cream has also been used postoperatively to aid wound healing; these reports are anecdotal and not found in the literature. Progressive increase in ambulation and activity is encouraged without pulling and separation of the wound edges. The patient is told to keep her legs closed or crossed at most times to reduce tension on the wound edges. The patient is seen 2 and 6 weeks after surgery.

The sutures start dissolving rapidly at approximately days 10 through 14. Significant itching and discharge may occur and can be reduced by placing diphenhydramine cream. Many patients interpret the discharge as an infection, but it usually is not. At week 4, the wound edges are typically closed well; bathing is allowed, and increased activity can be started. By week 6 to 8, the healing is complete, and no restrictions are needed. The patient can begin to have sex approximately 6 to 8 weeks after surgery, when the edges are

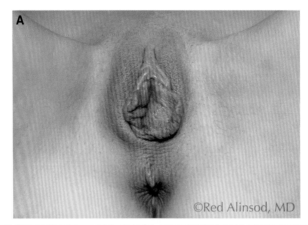

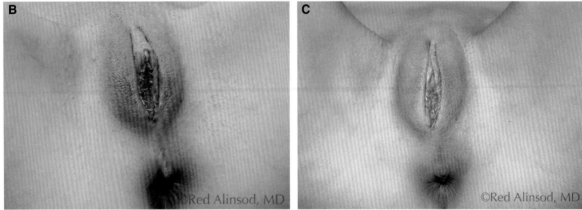

Fig. 5-7   A, Preoperative appearance. **B,** Immediately after surgery. **C,** Two-month postoperative result.

fully healed and softened. Results and outcomes are generally very favorable (Fig. 5-7), but a small percentage of women will require a revision surgery to smoothen uneven edges or reduce dog-ears.

Results and Outcomes

Many studies reveal a high level of satisfaction in women who undergo labia minora labiaplasty performed using various surgical techniques.[8] Of 177 patients who had labiaplasty and/or clitoral hood reduction, 97.2% were satisfied overall with the outcomes.[19] Trichot et al[27] conducted a retrospective evaluation of 21 patients who had a labiaplasty with either a pedicled flap reconstruction (86%) or a nymphectomy technique (14%). Of 18 survey respondents, all were satisfied with the results of the procedure (mean rating 8.7 of 10; 10 = highest rating).

Concurrent labia majora and minora reductions were performed safely and effectively, combined with clitoral hood reduction surgery, in more than 100 patients (6-year data).[4] In 2011 I demonstrated the benefits of the unified approach in a surgical video at the Congress on Aesthetic Vaginal Surgery.[4] Combination surgery was also reported to be safe and effective in two case reports.[22-25,27,28] Di Saia[28] reported on a patient who underwent a two-stage operation. The minora reduction was performed about 5 months after resolution of a postoperative hematoma that formed after the majora reduction. The patient was satisfied with the outcomes of both surgeries 6 weeks after the second stage of her treatment had been completed. More recently, Miklos and Moore[22] described subsequent surgical therapy in a patient with enlargement of both the labia minora and majora. For concurrent labia minoraplasty and majoraplasty surgery, I recommend performing the majoraplasty first to more accurately estimate the amount of remaining labia minora tissue needing excision.[3] After excision of the labia minora, the lateral labia tend to retract and pull the minora down; therefore performing the minoraplasty first may result in a greater loss of minora than ideally preferred.

Rezai and Jansson[9] conducted a comparative study of W-shaped resections of the protuberant tissue (50 patients) versus deepithelialized reduction labiaplasty (50 patients). Patients in both groups noted improvement in chronic irritations, sexual intercourse, and hygiene, and mitigation of their other main complaints in the 6-month postoperative review. Of the patients who underwent a W-shaped resection, 5 were dissatisfied with the appearance of the minora edge. In 8 patients, sensation did not return to the labia minora until up to 2 years after the operation. In another study of 21 patients who had an inferior wedge resection and a superior pedicle flap reconstruction, 95.2% were pleased with the outcomes of the surgery, whereas 85.7% viewed the aesthetic results as good or very good.[23]

Alter[17] performed an innovative central wedge reduction, usually concurrently with a lateral clitoral hood reduction, using the extension of the lateral hockey stick design in 407 patients. Of 166 patients who responded to his survey questionnaire, the average score was 9.2 of 10 (10 = most pleased), with improvement in self-esteem, sex life, and discomfort reported by 93%, 71%, and 95% of respondents, respectively. The complication rate was significantly low (4%), and 98% stated they would undergo the surgery again. Similarly, Solanki et al[15] observed favorable aesthetic and functional outcomes in 12 patients who underwent a reduction labiaplasty with the Maas and Hage technique of a running interdigitating W-shaped excision. One patient developed a painful hematoma 2 hours postoperatively, and one had urinary retention after surgery and required overnight catheterization. With the Maas and Hage technique, opposing Z-shaped incisions are closed with a tensionless zigzag suture line running obliquely across the edge of the labium. This surgical method decreases the likelihood of wound dehiscence and of advancement of the posterior fourchette, which can lead to tightening of the introitus. The patients were pleased with their natural-looking aesthetic outcomes and no revision surgeries were performed at 14 weeks postoperatively.[15]

Rouzier et al[26] conducted a study of 163 women who had a labial reduction operation. Ninety-eight patients returned their questionnaires. The satisfaction rate was 83% for the surgical outcomes overall, and 89% and 93% for cosmetic and functional results, respectively. Four patients (about 4%) stated that they would not undergo the same procedure again. Dehiscence occurred in 7% of cases. Surgeon experience and skill are of the utmost importance when performing wedge labiaplasties or linear resections, because, at least in my series,[4] most of the revisions were carried out on patients whose primary surgeons had performed a low volume of labiaplasties.

Problems and Complications

Adverse effects linked with labia minora reductions overall have been very low, ranging from 2.65%[10] to 4%[17,27] and 6%.[19] Complications associated with labiaplasties include postoperative infection,[9] hematoma,[5,8,15] infection, asymmetry, poor wound healing, premature suture absorption or breakage, undercorrection or overcorrection,[3,5] urinary retention,[3,5,15] skin retraction,[3] late local pain, and transient dyspareunia.[4,8] Dyspareunia occurred primarily when the labial suturing involved the introitus.[4] In a case report, the wedge excision technique was associated with postoperative complications of bleeding and transient hypersensitivity for 4 to 6 weeks after surgery.[27]

Flap techniques increase the risk of tissue necrosis,[1] whereas the type of suture may affect the risk of wound dehiscence.[8] A running absorbable rather than buried suture can lead to scalloping along the free border of the labia minora.[3,5] There are few statistics on revision surgeries of labiaplasties, but overcorrection and undercorrection potentially can occur in any labia minora reduction procedure.[16] Perhaps the most troublesome complication occurs when the entire labia minora is removed or the labia minora retracts more than expected, resulting in an inadvertent Barbie look in a patient who requested a rim or hybrid appearance.[4]

Studies of labia minora labiaplasties reveal high rates of overall satisfaction with cosmetic and functional results* and psychosocial outcomes, including improved self-esteem.[5,18,19,29] As new options for surgical technique become available, clinicians increasingly will have access to an armamentarium of multiple techniques that, if appropriate, may be combined in the same procedure. Although the edge excision technique reportedly has fewer wound-healing complications, it leaves a suture line at the periphery that may result in scar contracture and chronic pain during coitus.[2] These adverse effects are extremely rare, because the vulvovaginal complex is very forgiving and rarely scars for the long term.[4] Some experts consider the wedge resection the technique of choice,[25] whereas others view deepithelialized reduction as the standard of care.[9]

---

*References 5, 8, 9, 17, 19, 23, 26, 27.

Although there is no consensus on a procedural standard of care,[4] different techniques may be preferable for different patients. The technique chosen for each patient will depend on the advantages and disadvantages of the procedure, the degree and location of labia minora hypertrophy, and the patient's cosmetic preference. Some women prefer to preserve the dark, natural-looking edge of the labia minora and request only reduction of the labial bulk, whereas others want the edges removed.[2,3] Compared with other minora reduction procedures, RF labia minora labiaplasty offers increased safety, precision, function, and cosmesis when it is performed by a properly trained and experienced practitioner.[4] Future studies that incorporate principles of patient-centered medicine can shed light on the most effective surgical techniques for labia minora reductions based on patient characteristics and goals.

References

1. Mirzabeigi MN, Moore JH Jr, Mericli AF, et al. Current trends in vaginal labioplasty: a survey of plastic surgeons. Ann Plast Surg 68:125, 2012.
2. Ellsworth WA, Rizvi M, Lypka M, et al. Techniques for labia minora reduction: an algorithmic approach. Aesthetic Plast Surg 34:105, 2010.
3. Alinsod R. Overview of vaginal rejuvenation, new frontiers in pelvic surgery. Presented at the Annual Meeting of the National Society of Cosmetic Physicians and the American Academy of Cosmetic Gynecologists, Las Vegas, NV, Sept 2006.
4. Alinsod R. Awake in-office Barbie labiaplasty, awake in-office labia majora plasty, awake in-office vaginoplasty, awake in-office labial revision, sutureless band release, awake in-office mesh excision, labia majora Pellevé. Presented at the Congress on Aesthetic Vaginal Surgery, Tucson, AZ, Nov 2011.
5. Davison SP, West JE, Baker CL, et al. Medscape. Labiaplasty and labia minora reduction. Available at *http://emedicine.medscape.com/article/1372175-overview*.
6. Moore RD, Miklos JR. Vaginal reconstruction and rejuvenation surgery: is there data to support improved sexual function. Am J Cosmet Surg 29:97, 2012.
7. Giraldo F, González C, de Haro F. Central wedge nymphectomy with a 90-degree Z-plasty for aesthetic reduction of the labia minora. Plast Reconstr Surg 113:1820; discussion 1826, 2004.
8. Tepper OM, Wulkan M, Matarasso A. Labioplasty: anatomy, etiology, and a new surgical approach. Aesthet Surg J 31:511, 2011.
9. Rezai A, Jansson P. Clinical techniques: evaluation and result of reduction labioplasty. Am J Cosmet Surg 24, 2007. Available at *http://elitecosmeticsurgery.ae/wp-content/uploads/Article2.pdf*.
10. Felicio Yde A. Labial surgery. Aesthet Surg J 27:322, 2007.
11. Alter GJ. A new technique for aesthetic labia minora reduction. Ann Plast Surg 40:287, 1998.
12. Aleem S, Adams EJ. Labiaplasty. Obstet Gynaecol Reprod Med 22:50, 2012.
13. Choi HY, Kim KT. A new method for aesthetic reduction of labia minora (the deepithelialized reduction of labioplasty). Plast Reconstr Surg 105:419; discussion 423, 2000.
14. Hodgkinson DJ, Hait G. Aesthetic vaginal labioplasty. Aesthetic vaginal labioplasty. Plast Reconstr Surg 74:414, 1984.
15. Solanki NS, Tejero-Trujeque R, Stevens-King A, et al. Aesthetic and functional reduction of the labia minora using the Maas and Hage technique. J Plast Reconstr Aesthet Surg 63:1181, 2010.
16. Alter GJ. Labia minora reconstruction using clitoral hood flaps, wedge excisions, and YV advancement flaps. Plast Reconstr Surg 127:2356, 2011.
17. Alter GJ. Aesthetic labia minora and clitoral hood reduction using extended central wedge resection. Plast Reconstr Surg 122:1780, 2008.

18. Goodman MP. Female genital cosmetic and plastic surgery: a review. J Sex Med 8:1813, 2011.
19. Goodman MP, Placik OJ, Benson RH III, et al. A large multicenter outcome study of female genital plastic surgery. J Sex Med 7(4 Pt 1):1565, 2010.
20. Cao YJ, Li FY, Li SK, et al. A modified method of labia minora reduction: the de-epithelialised reduction of the central and posterior labia minora. J Plast Reconstr Aesthet Surg 65:1096, 2012.
21. Pardo J, Solà V, Ricci P, et al. Laser labioplasty of labia minora. Int J Gynaecol Obstet 93:38, 2016.
22. Miklos JR, Moore RD. Postoperative cosmetic expectations for patients considering labiaplasty surgery: our experience with 550 patients. Surg Technol Int 21:170, 2011.
23. Munhoz AM, Filassi JR, Ricci MD, et al. Aesthetic labia minora reduction with inferior wedge resection and superior pedicle flap reconstruction. Plast Reconstr Surg 118:1237, 2006.
24. Maas SM, Hage JJ. Functional and aesthetic labia minora reduction. Plast Reconstr Surg 105:1453, 2000.
25. Dobbeleir JM, Landuyt KV, Monstrey SJ. Aesthetic surgery of the female genitalia. Semin Plast Surg 25:130, 2011.
26. Rouzier R, Louis-Sylvestre C, Paniel BJ, et al. Hypertrophy of labia minora: experience with 163 reductions. Am J Obstet Gynecol 182(1 Pt 1):35, 2000.
27. Trichot C, Thubert T, Faivre E, et al. Surgical reduction of hypertrophy of the labia minora. Int J Gynaecol Obstet 115:40, 2011.
28. Di Saia JP. An unusual staged labial rejuvenation. J Sex Med 5:1263; discussion 1263, 2000.
29. Goodman MP. Female cosmetic genital surgery. Obstet Gynecol 113:154, 2009.

CHAPTER 6

Labia Majora Reduction Surgery: Majoraplasty

Red Alinsod

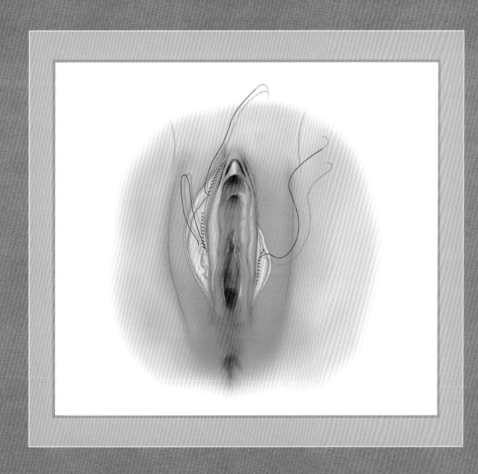

Key Points

- Labia majoraplasty is generally well tolerated and associated with favorable clinical outcomes.

- Removal of excess, loose skin does not appear to damage large vessels or nerves or affect sensitivity of the skin.

- Bleeding is an important potential complication when fat pad excision techniques are employed and larger deeper vessels are transected.

- Pain control is more challenging after fat pad removal.

- Preliminary findings suggest that high-frequency monopolar radiofrequency (RF) and standard electrocautery are beneficial surgical tools in labia majora reduction surgery.

- Labia minoraplasties and labia majoraplasties may be performed as staged operations in the same patient. When performed by surgeons with advanced training, a combined and unified approach to simultaneous labia minoraplasty and labia majoraplasty is practical and safe in selected patients.

The labia majora, composed largely of fatty tissue, are bilateral structures of the vulva that extend from the bottom of the mons pubis to the rectum.[1,2] Anatomic variation in the length and volume of the labia majora is normal and does not usually indicate a pathologic condition. The length is 7.0 to 12.0 cm, with a mean measurement of 9.3 cm.[3] Hereditary and environmental factors may contribute to individual variance in the size and shape of the labia majora. With a loss of volume, the labia majora may droop or sag with aging and after bariatric surgery[4,5] (Fig. 6-1). Excess fat deposits (genetic or from general obesity) can enlarge and stretch the labia majora. Prominent skin laxity of the labia majora in patients who have had significant weight loss can be quite astounding and distressing and may require RF shrinkage or surgical reduction.[6]

Prominent or bulky labia majora may be problematic for some women, typically by causing an embarrassing bulging under pants, swimsuits, and tight-fitting clothing.[6-8] They may lead to functional problems with sexual intercourse, poor hygiene, and physical discomfort in the genital region. Examples of those affected include bikers, horseback riders, and rowers who have chronic vulvar rubbing.[9,10] Some women have lowered self-esteem because of the undesirable physical appearance of their majora.[6] A common derogatory, slang term for hypertrophic and visually unappealing labia majora is *camel toes.*[9,10] Several websites unfairly highlight "camel toes" in young celebrities, which actually are normal and healthy

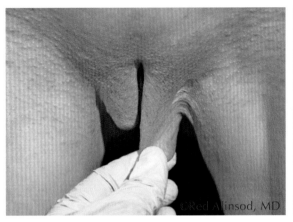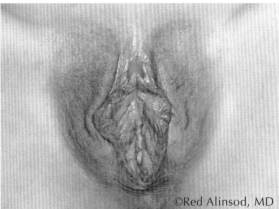

Fig. 6-1 The aging vulva and vagina. Bikini shaving, effects of gravity, and decreased collagen, elastin, and volume are contributing factors in the rise of labia majoraplasty surgery.

labia majora. However, some women are born with very prominent fat pads in the labia majora. Symptomatic labia majora issues that warrant medical attention are typically seen in middle-aged to older women but rarely in, for example, 21-year-old women.[10]

Indications and Contraindications

Labiaplasty is a plastic surgical procedure performed to reduce the size of hypertrophic labia, usually to improve the aesthetic appearance of the vulval area.[1,5,7,10-12] It involves removal of excess labia majora skin and prominent fat pads and is akin to a modified radical vulvectomy but without excision of groin lymph nodes. Rarely, this technique is employed to dramatically reduce the uncomfortable edema from congenital lymphedema of the vulva.[9] Labial reductions are typically performed on the labia minora and increasingly on the labia majora of female baby boomers, in whom aging often leads to sagging majora.[9] Primary labia majora hypertrophy results from volume excess from fat deposits, whereas secondary labia majora excess is caused by volume loss, leading to skin excess.[5,7]

Labia majoraplasty is performed for either aesthetic or functional purposes or both and less commonly than labia minoraplasty. Reduction of the majora tissue is indicated for patients with hypertrophic labia majora over a wide range of ages, and for those who have undergone substantial weight and fat loss with resultant majora laxity.[7,10] In affluent communities, such as the beach cities in the United States, the demand for labia majoraplasty is on par with the demand for labia minora reduction.[9,10]

Contraindications include undiagnosed vulvar lesions and vulvar dystrophies, active infectious lesions such as herpes and human papillomavirus. Relative contraindications include foreseen large-weight loss that may result in more skin laxity of the majora. Weight loss should preclude surgical labia majoraplasty.

Patient Evaluation

The patient is evaluated while she is in a lithotomy position and also while she is standing to best assess the anatomy involved and to confirm her desired, ideal appearance. The extent of the labia majora laxity is evaluated and photographed to help plan the surgical course of action. Markings may be placed to show looseness and asymmetry and the location of the suture lines. During the examination, the patient is given a mirror for visualizing the area to ensure she and the surgeon are discussing the same structures. The patient can point out the areas of concern and show how much tissue needs to be removed. By manually manipulating the labia majora, the surgeon can approximate the patient's desired postoperative appearance. The surgeon can explain that overly aggressive removal of labia majora tissue can result in pulling open of the lateral vaginal opening, creating a gaping vagina. Carefully asking whether this will be bothersome is essential. A more aggressive reduction can be performed in patients who do not mind a pulled-open appearance of the vaginal opening. However, less tissue removal is best for those concerned about the aesthetic appearance of the vaginal opening. Surgeons should stress that moderation is the goal for surgery.

A general physical examination and a pregnancy test in women in their reproductive years are recommended. Other blood work, such as a CBC and electrolytes, is typically not necessary in healthy women. Other specific tests can be ordered on a case-by-case basis.

Preoperative Planning and Preparation

After extensive discussions, the surgeon and patient agree on a plan, which is documented with drawings and/or photographs of how much tissue will be excised. Detailed consent is obtained once the patient has been screened and has clearly stated her desired amount of reduction of labia majora tissue.

Surgical Technique

Anesthesia

Patients are instructed to place a numbing cream (EMLA or compounded topical anesthetics) on the surgical sites approximately 2 hours before surgery. When labia majoraplasty is performed in the office, dermoelectroporation can be performed for 15 to 30 minutes to push the macromolecular numbing cream under the skin to provide comfort during the placement of local anesthesia. Approximately 10 ml of a local anesthetic with epinephrine should be prepared with the use of a 30-gauge needle to prevent over-distension of tissue. Oral or intramuscular narcotics are given in combination with an anxiolytic agent such as Valium or Ativan. A long-acting liposome-coated local anesthetic, such as Exparel, is ideal as an adjunct for postoperative pain control; this can last 72 hours or more. If Exparel is used, lidocaine must not be included, because it appears to break down the liposome and reduces the duration of effect of Exparel.

Markings

Fig. 6-2 shows typical markings. A vertical line is marked, beginning at the top level of the clitoral hood and extending in the labial crease, between the lateral labia majora and the medial clitoral hood and labia minora. The line is drawn down to the level of the introitus. A semielliptical mark is made from the top of the vertical line and extending laterally just past the top ridge of the labia majora, curving back down toward the lowest point of the vertical line. This is repeated on the opposite side for symmetry. Excising a moderate amount of labia majora tissue is recommended to prevent the appearance of a gaping vaginal opening, which occurs if excess labia majora is removed, as discussed previously.

Patient Positioning

The patient is placed in a low lithotomy position with adequate support of the legs to ensure comfort and good blood flow. Support under the knees and calf is recommended over simple heel support.

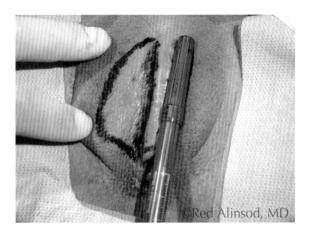

Fig. 6-2 Markings on the crease between the labia minora and labia majora are made with a standard medical skin marker. Hugging the curves and lines of the clitoral hood region and labia minora medially will help to better hide suture lines. Excess skin removal is advised.

Technique

Surgical equipment and modalities used in labia majora reduction include liposuction, scalpel-based excision, standard electrocautery, contact lasers, and RF excision. Liposuction may be used to treat volume excess of primary labia majora hypertrophy, but it may result in loose or uneven-hanging excess skin and lumpiness. Results from liposuction have been disappointing because of the limited amount of fat that can be extracted from the labia majora. Removal of the excess fat does not address the loose and excess skin. Most labia majoraplasties are performed to decrease the prominence and floppiness of redundant skin after volume loss. The liposuction procedure can be combined with labial reduction surgery but is not necessary if excisional labia majoraplasty is performed. Direct vaporization or excision of excess underlying fat is an advantage of excisional labia majoraplasty.[7,10] Furthermore, liposuction of the mons pubis or labia majora performed at the time of labial surgery may be problematic because of the pronounced edema and bruising of the labial tissues that can distort anatomy and create uneven healing.

In patients with volume excess, reduction may be achieved with fat excision with or without liposuction, skin excision, or both methods.[5,6] Because liposuction may produce sagging and excess skin, the established, older technique for labia majora reduction is preferred. It involves a vertical or modified, football-shaped wedge excision, starting on the top of the majora bilaterally and extending down toward the level of the perineum.[5] Excess tissue of the labia majora is removed using a vertical, football-shaped incision of the hypertrophic midportion with edge reanastamosis using fine absorbable sutures.[5,13] The incision is made along the length of the labia majora, at the top level of the clitoral hood complex, and down to the level of the introitus.[5,7,10] This procedure is often performed in the office with the patient under local anesthesia, and it is completed in 60 to 90 minutes. It results in a visible vertical scar on top of the labia majora that can be hidden if the patient maintains some pubic hair growth.

A sculpted linear resection with edge repair using layered monofilament suture material is a more refined and aesthetic approach.[7] In this alternative approach, a crescent-shaped medial inner portion of the labia majora is excised precisely on the crease between the minora and majora, with the excision directed upward just past the highest ridge of the labia majora.[7] The scar can be concealed in the crease between the inner and outer labia, providing a natural-looking result. Labia majoraplasty can be performed in either the operating room or the office with the patient under local anesthesia. Experienced labial surgeons can perform 98% of their labia minoraplasties and majoraplasties in the office with patients under local anesthesia.[9,10] This procedure is performed in approximately 60 to 90 minutes (Fig. 6-3). In this technique, RF pinpoint excision removes the marked labia majora tissue. The use of standard cautery, a CO_2 laser, or a 980-diode laser is acceptable, but these methods are less precise. Cold-knife excision is also acceptable. Once the edge incisions are made and the skin edges have been spared from eschar and burns,

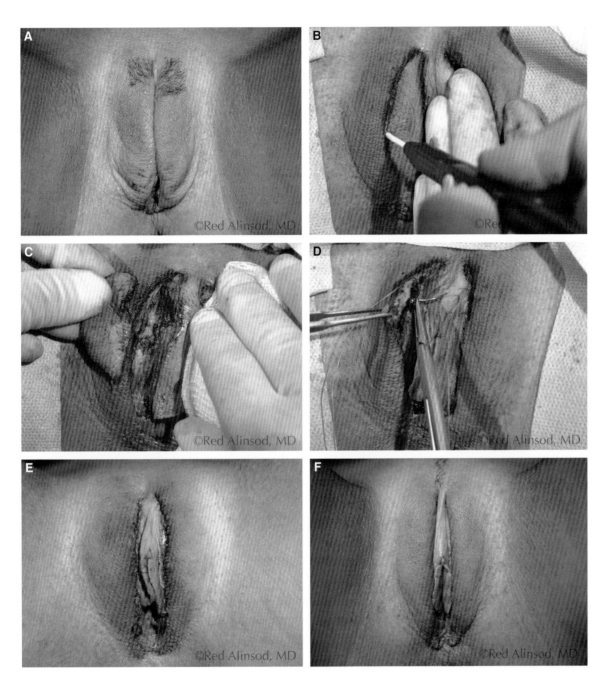

Fig. 6-3 Labia majoraplasty. **A,** Preoperative appearance. **B,** Excision. **C,** Hemostasis. **D,** Layered closure. **E,** Immediately after surgery. **F,** Two-month postoperative appearance. Labia majoraplasty tends to have more bruising of the surgical site, compared with labia minoraplasty. Ensuring complete hemostasis before skin closure is essential. The postoperative use of ice packs and cooling measures provides comfort and reduces bruising.

the underlying tissues are transected with standard cautery for hemostasis. Only a "skinning" excision is needed in most patients who do not have a large underlying fat pad. Usually, little fat is present beneath the labia majora skin, and white fascial tissue is immediately seen. A small percentage of patients have prominent fat that can be vaporized by RF or standard cautery to thin and tighten the underlying tissues. Even more rare is the need to break through the fascial plane to remove a large fat pad. This requires more local anesthesia and is easier to perform in a surgery center with the patient under general anesthesia, because the fat pads have an abundance of nerve endings that are difficult to manage in the office.

Unilateral or bilateral webbing between the labia majora and minora can be repaired during a labiaplasty on both the minora and majora.[1] In this unified approach, known as a *radical labiaplasty*, a majoraplasty can be combined with a clitoral hood reduction and minoraplasty.[9,10] Deepithelialization of the lateral clitoral hood can be combined with an additional resection technique such as a five-flap Z-plasty to correct redundant folding between the labia minora and the labia majora.[1] The technique necessitates careful attachment of the frenulum to the labia majora. Leaving the frenulum beneath the clitoris with adequate length of approximately 1 to 2 cm is crucial for a smooth transition from the clitoral hood to the frenulum and to the attachment with the majora. This method can flatten a prominent clitoral hood complex and make it less protruberant. Ellman RF devices (Ellman International, Hicksville, NY) have proved effective for use in labia majoraplasty, with minimal thermal damage and potentially accelerated healing. The precision of these devices is essential for working in the clitoral hood complex to prevent tissue and nerve damage. RF energy can also be used on the fat pads to shrink the bulkiness of the majora and on the lateral clitoral hood to smoothen and shrink the skin in a manner akin to a CO_2 laser burn.[9,10] This unified approach, which is referred to as *radical labiaplasty,* is performed only by the most experienced aesthetic vulvovaginal surgeons on properly screened and selected patients.

Tension-free edge closure is the most important part of surgery[9] (see Fig. 6-3, *D*). A multilayered approach is appropriate for closing open areas and dead space to prevent bruising, bleeding, abscesses, and wide scarring. The deepest layer can be closed by interrupted or by an inverted mattress running suture. The use of 3-0 or 4-0 delayed absorbable suture such as Monocryl is best to prevent rapid autolysis that sometimes occurs with Vicryl. Next, subcuticular suture of 4-0 or 5-0 delayed absorbable Vicryl or Monocryl is placed. Last, a layer of multiple interrupted 4-0 or 5-0 Vicryl sutures is placed to close all gaps and improve cosmesis. A Vicryl type of suture is best for the interrupted, outermost layer to prevent the poking sensation from the sharp Monocryl tips. Suture sites underneath the skin may heal firmly over the next 6 weeks. This can be softened over 2 to 4 weeks with daily massage and topical estrogens. It may take as long as 3 months for the suture line to soften.

Matlock developed another approach—a modified perineoplasty—to reduce the bulkiness of the loose labia majora skin.[7] The goal of this method is to pull down and flatten protruberant labia majora to provide a more youthful-appearing vaginal opening with a V shape, instead of a U shape, at the bottom of the introitus. Overtightening may require correction with a sutureless band release.[9,10] Some plastic surgeons have used a complementary approach to pull the labia majora upward by performing a mons puboplasty or a modified abdominoplasty with upward traction to reduce the appearance of bulkiness in the vulvovaginal area. These procedures are best done before a labia majoraplasty to facilitate a more accurate evaluation of the amount of tissue reduction of the labia majora. Liposuction of the mons is ideally performed later in a separate procedure because of the extensive edema that develops in the mons down to the labia majora.

Ancillary Procedures

Ancillary procedures that can be performed during a labia majoraplasty include perineoplasty, turning a U-shaped introitus into a V-shaped introitus for a more youthful appearance. The downside of this approach is the potential for short-term, painful intercourse at the introitus. A labia minoraplasty and clitoral hood reduction can be performed after a labia majoraplasty. A labia majoraplasty is best performed first, followed by a labia minoraplasty and then a clitoral hood reduction for proper evaluation for symmetry and the degree of minora reduction. Labia majora reductions tend to have a pulling effect on the labia minora and flatten them somewhat. If the minora are reduced first, a labia majoraplasty surgery can accentuate the reduction of the minora. A requested moderate labial reduction may appear as a more radical reduction of labial tissue, because the pulling of the labia minora edges makes them look smaller or almost invisible in some cases.

Postoperative Care

Routine postoperative care instructions are reviewed. Patients are instructed not to place tension on the labia majora suture line to prevent premature suture breakage or a wound breakdown. They are advised to keep their legs together and to not spread them open widely. Walking in moderation is allowed, but gym activities, bike riding, horseback riding, and any sport causing pressure on the surgical edges are not. The use of cooling measures such as ice packs is advised for comfort and to reduce swelling. Placing an ice pack on the site (20 minutes on and 20 minutes off continually for the first few days up to 1 week) may be ideal.

Daily hygiene and care of the surgical site involve washing with mild soap and water and dabbing dry. Patients should not rub the areas, swim, bathe, or sit in standing water such as Sitz baths. Soaking tends to weaken sutures prematurely. Daily postoperative estradiol cream placed on the labia and over the wound sites is advised to aid healing and prevent clothing from adhering to the surgical site. Empiric use of estrogen vaginal cream may help with healing and comfort, but no controlled studies have been done to prove its superiority over the use of no creams. Some surgeons advocate placing collagen cream to aid in wound healing. These results are anecdotal in the literature. Postoperative antibiotics have been used widely after vaginal surgery, but no consensus on duration and type has been reported. Most infections that occur are urinary in origin. If an antibiotic is deemed necessary, a wide-spectrum antibiotic is recommended for 7 to 10 days postoperatively. Patients are seen again 2 and 6 weeks after surgery. Normal activities, including exercise and sex, are typically approved at 6 to 8 weeks postoperatively.

Results and Outcomes

Di Saia[14] performed a cosmetic reduction of the labia minora and labia majora in a 42-year-old woman seeking aesthetic modification of her vulvar region. He planned a two-stage reduction operation, starting with a labia majora reduction. The patient developed a postoperative hematoma that was subsequently evacuated. Hypersensitivity in the exposed area of her genitalia resolved in 4 to 6 weeks. A labia minoraplasty was performed 4 months later, and 6 weeks postoperatively the patient was satisfied with the results of the procedure. In a separate, rare case report, Miklos and Moore[15] performed concurrent labiaplasties of the minora and majora in a woman presenting with hypertrophy of the labia minora and labia majora. The surgeries were deemed effective and safe with no serious complication.

In my series reported in 2011, 100 women with an average age of 45 years who underwent the curved linear approach and my unified technique reported 98% satisfaction and no serious complications.[9] Two patients were not satisfied with the outcomes and requested removal of additional tissue in a second labia majoraplasty. The procedure was again performed and both patients were extremely satisfied with the postoperative results. Two patients required resuturing but showed no evidence of infections and had an average blood loss of 10 ml. All procedures in this series were performed in the office on awake patients. No intravenous access was needed, and all medications were given as a cream, orally, or by intramuscular injection. The patient self-hydrated by sipping water through the entire case. The average total volume of local anesthesia used was 4 ml for labia minoraplasty, 7 ml for labia majoraplasty, and 15 ml for the unified approach. More bleeding occurred (50 to 100 ml) when significant fat pad removal was performed. No long-term dyspareunia was reported. No adverse anesthetic effects occurred except for the rare and transient vasovagal response after surgery when the procedure was done in the afternoon hours. These patients were deemed *volume low* and responded well with oral fluid intake.[9]

Generally, patient satisfaction is high and surgical complications are low with labia majoraplasty. In my series, wound breakdown and the need for revision surgery was lower with labia majoraplasty compared with labia minoraplasty. Patients commonly reported an increase in comfort and self-confidence because of a reduction in self-awareness of the prominent labia majora. Results can be aesthetically dramatic when labia majora surgery is combined with labia minora surgery and a vaginoplasty/perineoplasty (Figs. 6-4 and 6-5) and when large fat pads are excised (Figs. 6-6 and 6-7).

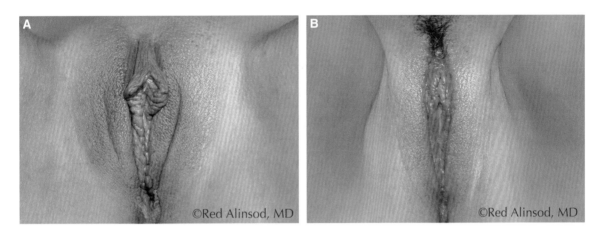

Fig. 6-4 This is an example of a combined labia minoraplasty and labia majoraplasty surgery. **A,** Preoperative appearance. **B,** Two-month postoperative result.

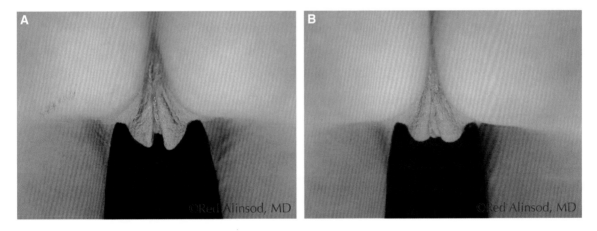

Fig. 6-5 This patient underwent reduction of the large and prominently loose labia majora, with a resultant youthful look as seen from behind, a view most helpful in showing what partners see. **A,** Preoperative appearance. **B,** Two-month postoperative result.

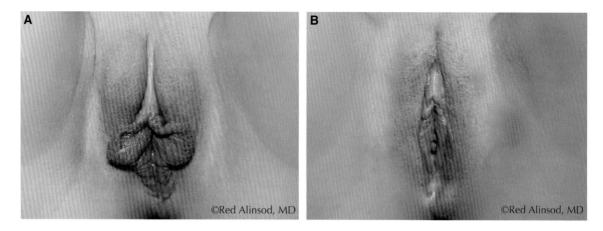

Fig. 6-6 A, Preoperative appearance. **B,** Two-month postoperative result.

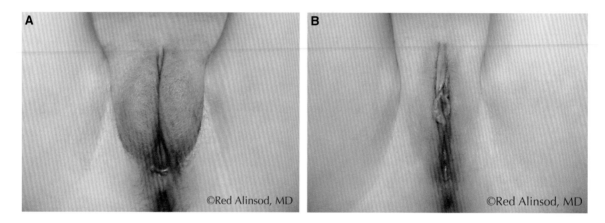

Fig. 6-7 A, Preoperative appearance before fat pad removal. **B,** Two-month postoperative result.

Problems and Complications

Postoperative complications associated with labial excision include mild to moderate pain, bleeding, bruising, transient edema, and transient hypersensitivity for 4 for 6 weeks.[5,14] Ice packs and oral narcotics help to reduce the edema and discomfort. The average blood loss for labia majoraplasty is 5 to 10 ml.[9] The bleeding complication Di Saia[14] observed after stage one of a two-stage labiaplasty did not lead to delayed wound healing or distortion. In my series the most common complication was premature suture breakage in 5% of patients from physical activity that pulled the edges apart, thereby necessitating resuturing. Strict adherence to a tension-free healing regimen of approximately 4 to 6 weeks is crucial.[9] Tying the interrupted sutures too tightly can result in scalloping of the surgical edges, with visible horizontal lines. This is worsened if significant edema causes the skin to expand against a tight suture. Pubic hair growth extending up to the crease between the minora and majora is potentially irritating and may need treatment. Laser/intense pulsed light hair reduction treatments can control this problem in those who do not shave their vulva. This is not a problem for women who regularly shave or wax their vulva.[7]

References

1. Davison SP, West JE, Baker CL, et al. Medscape. Labiaplasty and labia minora reduction. Available at *http://emedicine.medscape.com/article/1372175-overview.*
2. Moore RD, Miklos JR. Vaginal reconstruction and rejuvenation surgery: is there data to support improved sexual function. Am J Cosmet Surg 29:97, 2012.
3. Lloyd J, Crouch NS, Minto CL, et al. Female genital appearance: "normality" unfolds. BJOG 112:643, 2005.
4. Salgado CJ, Tang JC, Desrosiers AE III. Use of dermal fat graft for augmentation of the labia majora. J Plast Reconstr Aesthet Surg 65:267, 2012.
5. Dobbeleir JM, Landuyt KV, Monstrey SJ. Aesthetic surgery of the female genitalia. Semin Plast Surg 25:130, 2011.
6. Alter GJ. Management of the mons pubis and labia majora in the massive weight loss patient. Aesthet Surg J 29:432, 2009.
7. Alinsod R. Overview of vaginal rejuvenation, new frontiers in pelvic surgery. Presented at the Annual Meeting of the National Society of Cosmetic Physicians and the American Academy of Cosmetic Gynecologists, Las Vegas, NV, Oct 2006.
8. Felicio AY. Labial surgery. Aesthet Surg J 27:322, 2007.
9. Alinsod R. Awake in-office Barbie labiaplasty, awake in-office labia majora plasty, awake in-office vaginoplasty, awake in-office labial revision, sutureless band release, awake in-office mesh excision, labia majora Pellevé. Presented at the Congress on Aesthetic Vaginal Surgery, Tucson, AZ, Nov 2011.
10. Alinsod R. Radical labia majora plasty, RF for labia majora laxity, surgical management of the camel toe, the unified approach to labiaplasty, awake in-office vaginoplasty, awake in-office labial revision. Presented at the Congress on Aesthetic Vaginal Surgery, Las Vegas, NV, Oct 2012.
11. Goodman M. Female genital cosmetic and plastic surgery: a review. J Sex Med 8:1813, 2011.
12. Goodman MP, Placik OJ, Benson RH III, et al. A large multicenter outcome study of female genital plastic surgery. J Sex Med 7(4 Pt 1):1565, 2010.
13. Goodman MP. Female cosmetic genital surgery. Obstet Gynecol 113:154, 2009.
14. Di Saia J. An unusual staged labial rejuvenation. J Sex Med 5:1263, 2008.
15. Miklos JR, Moore RD. Postoperative cosmetic expectations for patients considering labiaplasty surgery: our experience with 550 patients. Surg Technol Int 21:170, 2001.

CHAPTER 7

Clitoral Hood Reduction Techniques

Otto J. Placik

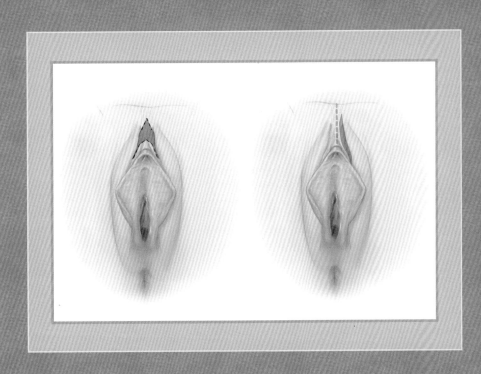

Key Points

- *Clitoral hood reduction (CHR) is rarely performed as an isolated procedure.*

- *CHR is most commonly performed in combination with labia minora reduction.*

- *Functional outcomes of CHR are poorly understood, and the effect on sexual function has not been established.*

- *CHR is typically more of an aesthetic procedure.*

- *CHR should be distinguished from clitoral procedures.*

- *The procedure is not female genital mutilation, infibulation, cultural/ritualistic female circumcision, or genital piercing.*

Indications and Contraindications

General Considerations

CHR is a procedure that is often confounded with clitoral hood removal, clitoroplasty, clitoral unhooding, clitoral hoodectomy, clitoropexy, hoodoplasty, dorsal slit surgery, lysis of adhesions, and unhooding. Understanding the difference between the glans/corpora clitoris and the prepuce is essential for distinguishing procedures. In the context of this chapter, the hood is the prepuce of the clitoris and is analogous to the penile foreskin. I intentionally do not use the term *circumcision,* because it has negative connotations and is often confused with clitoral amputation. The hood is distinctly different from the clitoris, and I will refer to CHR exclusively without focusing on clitoral surgery. Information on the surgery and its sequelae is sparce; a literature search on CHR yielded only 13 results. Part of the difficulty is that CHR is rarely performed as an isolated procedure and in most instances is performed in combination with labia minora reduction. CHR is predominantly performed for aesthetic indications and is limited to skin resection. Other procedures performed on the clitoris proper include the following:
- Clitoropexy to retract or suspend the clitoris
- Clitoral reduction (reduction clitoroplasty) to reduce the size of the clitoris, which most commonly occurs with congenital adrenal hyperplasia, ambiguous genitalia, female pseudohermaphroditism, clitoromegaly, clitoral hypertrophy, and genital virilism
- Clitoral lysis of adhesions, usually resulting from lichen sclerosus

In these operations, portions of the clitoral hood may be removed as an integral part of the reconstructive procedure, as discussed by Graves et al[1] for clitoral reduction and Ostrzenski[2] for buried clitoris. CHR should be further differentiated from female genital mutilation procedures, including infibulation and cultural or ritualistic female circumcision. Although genital piercing is often performed on the clitoral hood, it does not reduce the bulk of soft tissue.

Anatomic Issues

Although practitioners of aesthetic female genital surgery have an innate appreciation for the boundaries and extent of the clitoral hood, it is poorly defined in the literature. Some authors have referred to the hood (preputium clitoridis) as the *superior portion or division of the labia minora.*[3] The clitoral hood varies greatly among individuals, with either a smooth or irregularly folded/pleated surface, and is commonly asymmetrical.[4] Most anatomists refer to the free edge of the prepuce as the *clitoral hood.* Aesthetic surgeons consider the hood as extending anteriorly and superiorly to the anterior labial commissure (apex of the intervulvar cleft). The inferior border is the free edge of the prepuce and extends down to the junction with the labia minora. This serves as the defining point of the clitoral frenulum, the portion of the labia minora that extends to the clitoris and begins medial to the attachment with the clitoral hood. Some authors think the clitoral frenulum anchors and stabilizes the inferior attachment of the clitoral hood, and failure to respect this landmark may produce a clitoral hood deformity when a labiaplasty is performed.[5]

Laterally, the hood is bounded by the interlabial sulcus (Fig. 7-1). The length of the hood is measured from the anterior labial commissure to the distal prepuce, in the midline, and ranges from 2 to 6 cm.[4] Protrusion of the hood beyond the labia majora is not consistent

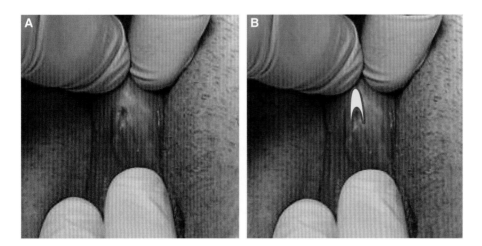

Fig. 7-1   A, The clitoral hood skin is retracted, exposing the clitoris and clitoral frenulum. **B,** The typical extent of the clitoral hood *(red).*

Continued

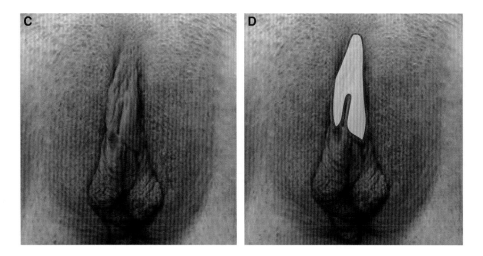

Fig. 7-1, cont'd   C, The same patient is shown in a lithotomy position without the clitoral hood skin retracted. **D,** The area addressed with CHR is outlined in *red*.

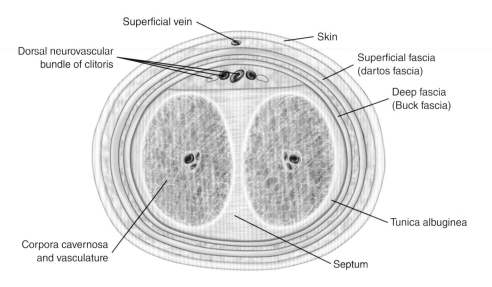

Fig. 7-2   A transverse section through the body of the clitoris.

and will vary with the size of the clitoris, with some resembling a small penis. The thickness is a function of the skin quality and the underlying subcutaneous tissue and dartos fascia. The layers of the midportion of the hood from superficial to deep are the skin, subcutaneous tissue, dartos fascia, Buck fascia and suspensory ligament, neurovascular bundle, tunica albuginea, and clitoris (Fig. 7-2).

An "ideal" configuration and relation of the glans clitoris to the prepuce has not been established. Typically, the glans clitoris will protrude slightly beyond the clitoral hood with varying degrees of visibility. Excessive prominence of the clitoral hood either in untreated or iatrogenic cases after isolated labiaplasty has been described as a "micropenis."[6]

The innervation of the clitoris and hood is generally attributed to the dorsal nerve of the clitoris, which crosses the perineal membrane 2.4 to 3.0 cm lateral to the urethral meatus (Fig. 7-3). It passes along the perineal membrane for 1.8 to 2.2 cm to the ischiopubic ramus, where it transitions to the anterolateral surface of the clitoral body, deep to the Buck fascia, for 2.0 to 2.5 cm.[7] Surgeons must use caution when dissecting deep to the Buck fascia and lateral to the midline over the clitoral hood and minimize surgery in the depths of the interlabial sulcus at the level of the meatus. Although anatomic studies in humans are limited, we know that the undersurface of the prepuce has many sensory nerves; any surgery on these tissues is discouraged unless indicated for such conditions as lichen sclerosus.[8]

The function of the prepuce is unknown but is purported to protect the clitoris and the eccrine glands, which, unique to females, keep the glandopreputial sulcus moistened.[9]

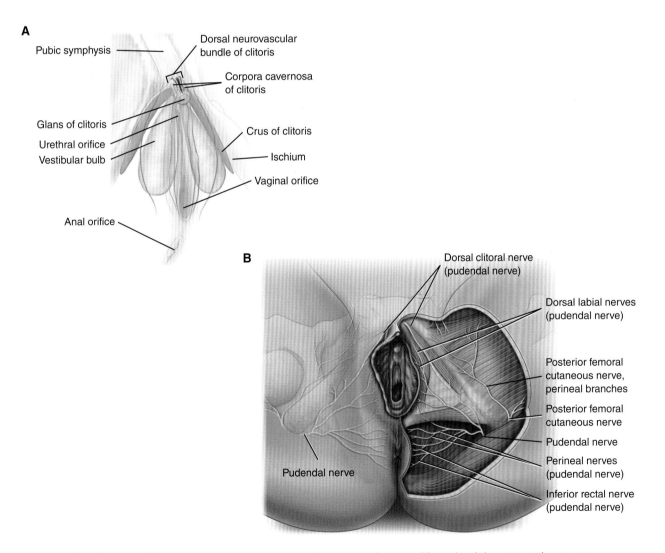

Fig. 7-3 **A,** Clitoral structures and relationship to pubic bones with pudendal nerve and sensory branches of the clitoris. **B,** Sensory nerves of the vulva and relationship to pelvic floor muscles.

Indications

The goals of surgery are to debulk and reduce the excess or redundant clitoral prepuce. However, the specific indications are less clear. Hodgkinson and Hait[10] reported that "aesthetic external genital surgery may be requested by females who feel that their sexual enjoyment will be enhanced by exposing the clitoris . . . or a reduction in size of the clitoris may be aesthetically more appealing."[10] However, their described procedure accomplished neither of these goals. Alter[11] later modified their description, stating that the "aesthetic ideal is labia minora and a clitoral hood that do not protrude past the labia majora." He referred to the elective nature of the procedure when noting that the surgery is "to excise redundant lateral labium and excess lateral clitoral hood (if desired by the patient)." Elsewhere he stated that the "excision allows for elimination of much of the unsightly lateral hood, which is a major aesthetic and often functional concern" but did not specify the initial functional impairment for which correction was sought or achieved.[12] Gress[13] reported that "the aim of the surgical procedures is to achieve a result that best fulfills the wishes and expectations of the patients" and is "as balanced as possible." Goodman[14] noted that CHR is intended "to produce more 'exposure' of the clitoral body, theoretically providing improved sexual stimulation" but did not substantiate this claim; he restated the aesthetic indications. de Alencar Felicio[6] stated that with CHR "the clitoris is exposed"; in a letter to the editor, Hunter[15] expressed his disagreement with this and stated that surgeons should "never expose/further expose the clitoris." Hamori[16] reported that findings that respond to CHR include projection beyond the labia majora or sufficient hood bulkiness that "exceeds the width of either surrounding labium majus" or "widening of the intervulvar commissure [anterior vulvar commissure]." She discussed patients' requests for a "petite labia minora and clitoral hood," but she also cautioned that "care must be taken . . . as this may cause exposure of the glans clitoris."[5]

Ostrzenski[17] distinguished between an elongated hood and a thickened hood. An elongated hood is treated to result in 3 to 5 mm of glans exposure using his earlier "hydrodissection with reverse V-plasty."[2] Patients were initially managed with a V-plasty for reasons of embarrassment: "feeling different and unhappy in an intimate relationship" and "noticeable overgrowing"; hygiene issues: "offensive odor," discomfort, elongation, a negative body image perception "responsible for her deterioration of social and emotional well-being"; and aesthetic correction of a "significantly protruding clitoral prepuce."[17]

The degree of exposure of the glans clitoris (3 to 5 mm) and the ability to improve sexual stimulation by diminishing tissue interference are controversial.[17] Benson[18] discussed the patients he thought would be happy with the procedure (Table 7-1). The issues of improved cosmetic appearance, contour, and folds are less debated.[14]

Table 7-1 Patients Likely To Be Satisfied With a Clitoral Hood Reduction Procedure

Will Likely Be Satisfied	Will Likely Not Be Satisfied
Anorgasmic Patients These patients will be happier with coitus even if no climax is achieved, if emotionally stable. Surgery is avoided if untreated emotional issues are evident.	**Patients With These Characteristics** These patients desire orgasm in the missionary position. These patients desire orgasm with no other stimulation except intercourse.
Orgasm Is Slow or Weak These patients are usually the most likely to be pleased with the result of the procedure; as intensity increases, speed to climax is variable.	**Currently Happy and Normal** Surgery is avoided unless a physical examination supports correction.
Orgasmic but Requires Manual/Oral/Vibrator/Positioning Patients will be pleased with increased sensation but will likely require extra stimulation.	**Low Sex Drive** If the condition has a psychological or hormonal basis, surgery will not help; the underlying condition must first be treated.
Painful Clitoris Pain may resolve when chronic infection or adhesions are treated.	**Seeking Multiorgasmic Status** Surgery on these patients is avoided; this result may occur but cannot be promised or necessarily delivered.
Labiaplasty Patients Patients will be pleased with a more contoured appearance.	**Menopausal Agglutination** Problems will recur if hormonal status is not normalized.
	Lichen Sclerosus Scarring This condition almost always recurs within a few months.
	Body Modifiers Surgery is not performed on these patients; they may not be satisfied with the results, and procedures may be difficult to reverse.

Adapted from Benson R. Clitoral hood reduction. Presented at the Seventh Annual Congress for Aesthetic Vaginal Surgery, Tucson, AZ, Jan 2012.

Nearly anyone who presents with realistic expectations and has excess preputial tissue is a candidate for an elective procedure. Several authors have described an iatrogenic clitoral hood deformity after labiaplasty."[5,11,13] Hamori[5] reported that the trim method of labia reduction may produce a relative reduction in the prominence of the labia minora in comparison to the residual clitoral hood with the excessive projection of the clitoral hood creating the illusion of a "small penis." However, she did not comment on whether a clitoral hood reduction was performed as part of the initial procedure, as is typically routine in most instances of labia reduction (R. Alinsod, personal communication, 2013). This may also occur as the result of an isolated labia reduction with the wedge technique (also called with inferior wedge resection and superior pedicle flap reconstruction), leading Dr. Alter[11,12] to modify his technique and rename it the *extended* central wedge resection. He stated that the extension was required to "excise the . . . excess lateral clitoral hood (if desired by the patient)."[12] In his discussion, Alter commented that the trim technique may result in an "abrupt-ending clitoral frenulum and large overhanging clitoral hood." The clitoral hood resection was described as either being continuous with the central wedge resection or, alternatively, as a discontinuous "separate elliptical excision." See Fig. 10-18 in Chapter 10 (Complications of Female Cosmetic Genital Surgery) for more information about this condition.

Contraindications

Contraindications to CHR include a patient's unrealistic expectations or comorbid untreated psychosexual conditions that may interfere with sexual function; patient confusion with hoodectomy procedures; active vulvovaginal infections; active vulvovaginal inflammatory diseases; coagulopathy; and smoking.

Patient Evaluation

Clinical Evaluation of the Deformity

Although screening methods for patients undergoing female genital plastic surgery have been recommended, including traditional assessments and sexual function surveys (particularly orgasmic dysfunction), no established tools for evaluating CHR candidates have been established. Because the surgery is rarely performed as an isolated procedure, evaluation typically proceeds as for a candidate for labia minora reduction. Hamori[5,16] suggested that clitoral hood redundancy is optimally assessed with the patient in the standing position, with attention to tissue thickness and bulk, redundant folds, symmetry, separation of the anterior vulvar commissure, and previous surgery (especially trim labiaplasty); the clitoris is also palpated to exclude clitoromegaly. Because Gress's technique[13] may affect the prominence of the clitoris, he suggested preoperative analysis of the clitoral glans and body to distinguish the hypertrophy of the glans from that of the hood, as well as the degree of "protrusion of the tip of the clitoris." He advised measuring the distance from the glans clitoris to the urethral meatus and stated that this must be a minimum of 1.5 cm.

Freedom of the prepuce from the glans clitoris and the presence of adhesions, phimosis, scars, piercings, trauma, pain, and dysesthesias should be documented. Lichen sclerosus should be excluded. The clitoris and prepuce have no standard appearance, and a wide variety of anatomic variations have been described.[19] Ostrzenski[20] proposed a clitoral hood classification that is not widely used but is most applicable to his described surgical approaches: occlusion as seen in lichen sclerosus (type 1), hypertrophy (type 2), and hypertrophy with subdermal asymmetry (type 3).

Preoperative Planning and Preparation

As with all surgical planning, a survey of patient motivations with counseling is an essential component of treatment.[21] After a complete history is taken and a physical examination completed, including psychological, gynecologic, and sexual evaluations, some practitioners advise that patients be referred for counseling with appropriate specialist management, such as cognitive behavioral therapy.[22] The assessment of sexual function is as important as the aesthetic and anatomic evaluation.[23] The Society of Obstetricians and Gynaecologists of Canada has suggested encouraging girls younger than 16 years of age to defer surgery until completion of mature genital development.[21] Patients should be informed about the procedure with a thorough review of the risks, alternatives, and benefits, consistent with the principles of informed consent.

When discussing the role and goals of the procedure, physicians should inform patients that the *normal* physical appearance is highly variable, and repair probably has no direct medical benefit. Patients' natural asymmetries and functional anatomy are reviewed.

Surgical Technique

A Brief History

In most texts, the technique is vaguely described and traditionally considered an adjunct to labia minora reduction. Historically, with treatment of clitoromegaly, portions of the clitoral hood have been removed as an integral part of clitoral reduction techniques[1] (Figs. 7-4 and 7-5).

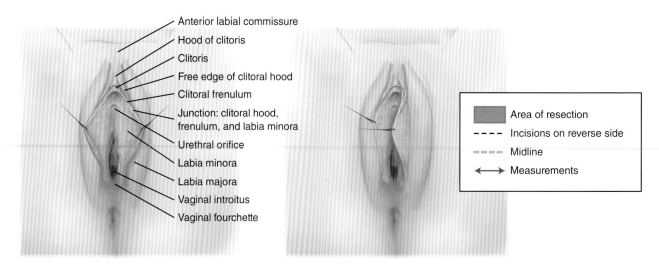

Anterior labial commissure
Hood of clitoris
Clitoris
Free edge of clitoral hood
Clitoral frenulum
Junction: clitoral hood, frenulum, and labia minora
Urethral orifice
Labia minora
Labia majora
Vaginal introitus
Vaginal fourchette

	Area of resection
----	Incisions on reverse side
====	Midline
⟷	Measurements

Fig. 7-4   Female vulvar anatomy.

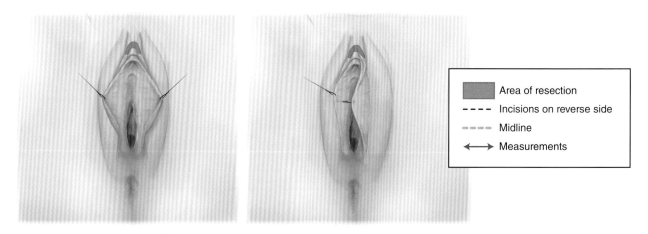

	Area of resection
----	Incisions on reverse side
====	Midline
⟷	Measurements

Fig. 7-5   CHR described by Graves et al[1] as an integral part of clitoromegaly surgery.

For aesthetic indications, the procedures were only recently reported. In 2005 Alter[24] first described his technique of combined labial wedge resection with the addition of a "lateral V excision curving up along the lateral clitoral hood to eliminate the dog-ear and, if desired, to excise redundant lateral clitoral hood skin. No lateral subcutaneous tissue is excised" (Fig. 7-6). Addressing the clitoral hood component was a modification of his previously reported technique, which accomplished isolated labia minora reduction only.[25] In 2006 Gress[26] provided the first illustration and photographic documentation using his so-called composite reduction labiaplasty, which combined reduction of labial tissue both above and below the clitoris using a modification of the trim or edge resection technique (Fig. 7-7).

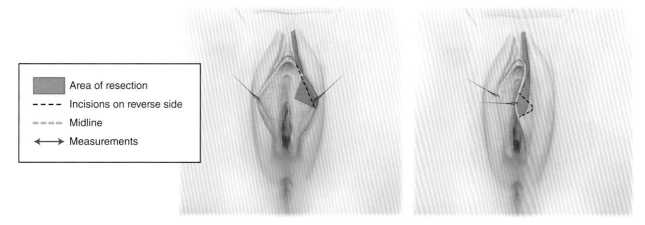

Fig. 7-6   CHR described by Alter[24] as an addition to labia minora wedge resection.

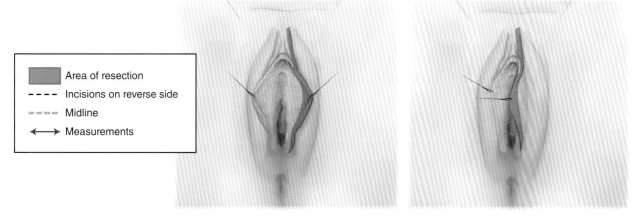

Fig. 7-7   CHR initially described by Gress[26] as part of a composite reduction labiaplasty.

In 2007 and 2008 Alter clarified his new technique in which the inner, medial wedge is designed essentially horizontally and over the central portions of the labia to remove the most "objectionable" projecting portion; the outer, lateral "wedge excision should then be curved laterally and anteriorly (hockey-stick) to excise this redundant lateral labium and excess lateral clitoral hood (if desired by the patient)."[12] "Therefore the internal and external V excisions are shaped differently, with the intervening subcutaneous tissue preserved while the leading labial edge is precisely reapproximated."[11] "Only enough tissue is excised to produce a good cosmetic result. This allows a better subcutaneous closure, which is necessary to prevent wound dehiscence and fistula formation."[12] In 2007 de Alencar Felicio[6] first discussed isolated CHR performed with a "fusiform excision lateral to the clitoris in each side" (Fig. 7-8). She stressed the importance of maintaining the midline orientation of the clitoris and a symmetrical design relative to the labia minora and majora and of achieving clitoral exposure (unspecified). However, she discouraged simultaneous labia minora reduction and CHR because of "prolonged edema."

In 2008 Apesos et al[27] described an inverted-V or chevronlike resection located high and directly over the center of the clitoral hood, with the apex located at the superior extent of the anterior labial commissure (Fig. 7-9). Advocates think this may help to "close" the gap between the labia majora, when present, in the anterior labial commissure. In 2013 Gress[13] further refined his original technique with the excision of a transverse crescent of tissue below the clitoris but above the urethral meatus that, when combined with the earlier description of the composite reduction labiaplasty, corrected clitoral protrusion (Fig. 7-10). Hamori[5] provided two approaches to CHR in her paper on postoperative clitoral hood deformities. The first is a resection of excess clitoral hood skin employing an inverted-V pattern over the dorsum of the clitoris. Unlike the placement used by

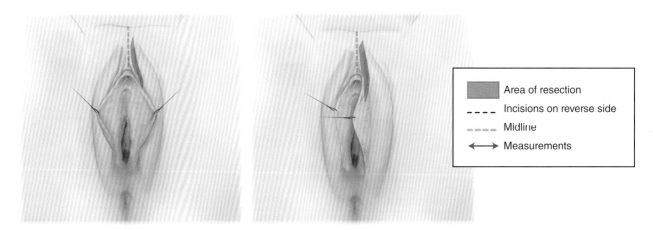

	Area of resection
_ _ _ _	Incisions on reverse side
_ _ _ _	Midline
←——→	Measurements

Fig. 7-8 Isolated CHR described by de Alencar Felicio.[6]

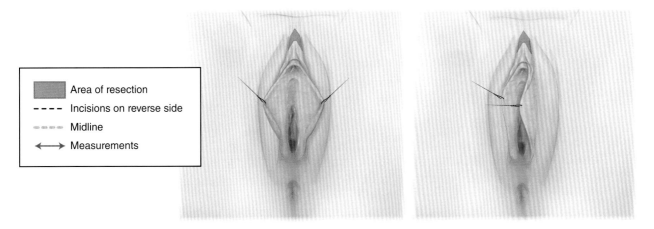

Fig. 7-9 Isolated CHR described by Apesos et al.[27]

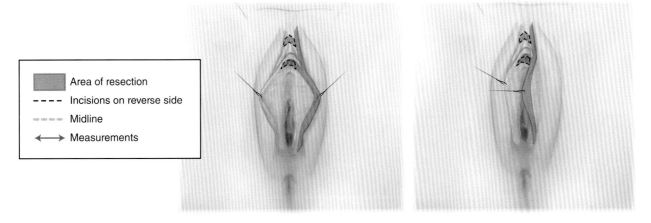

Fig. 7-10 CHR modification to treat clitoral protrusion, described by Gress[13] as part of a composite reduction labiaplasty.

Apesos et al,[27] the resection is centered low on the clitoral hood and is more similar to the location described by Graves et al[1] for the treatment of clitoromegaly (see Fig. 7-5). Conservative tissue removal is emphasized to minimize the potential for exposure of the glans. Other surgeons, such as de Alencar Felicio,[6] have noted this precaution, without an explanation of the adverse consequences. However, Triana and Robledo[28] explained that excessive protrusion may be associated with chronic "pain and discomfort while walking and sitting."

Hamori's second method[5] involves two paramedian lenticular excisions of the clitoral hood, parallel to the long axis of the body of the clitoris, intended to reduce "width rather than dorsal skin excess." This is similar to de Alencar Felicio's technique (see Fig. 7-8).

Very little documentation exists on the most popular of these techniques. From a personal survey, I have found that most practitioners use this latter approach and design the anterior limbs of the resection so that they diverge superiorly, a pattern that resembles an X or)(. However, a few surgeons prefer the incisions to converge superiorly to treat vertical redundancy, which appears more like a long inverted V or /\. Others use a transverse limb that looks like an H or)-(to shorten a vertically long hood (Fig. 7-11). Other modifica-

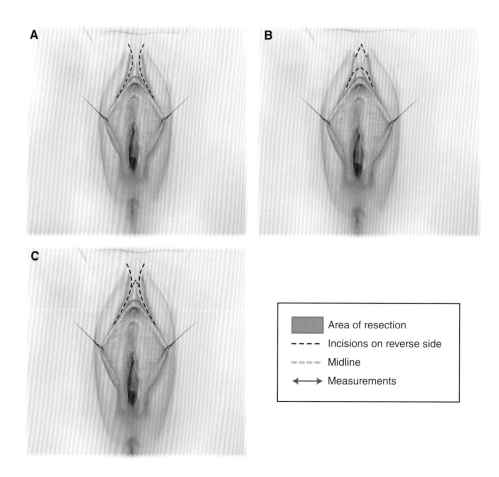

	Area of resection
- - - -	Incisions on reverse side
═ ═ ═ ═	Midline
⟷	Measurements

Fig. 7-11   Patterns of CHR. **A,**)(pattern. **B,** Inverted-V pattern. **C,** H pattern.

tions have been reported but were not well described, including the "horseshoe" resection Triana and Robledo[28] attributed to Kalra. The issues to address are the presence of vertical (length) and/or horizontal (width) excess and the degree of asymmetry. A thorough assessment of patients' relevant anatomy and treatment goals will guide surgeons in choosing the optimal approach to the clitoral hood.

My Technique: Anesthesia, Antibiotics, and Markings

CHR is rarely performed as an isolated procedure and most commonly accompanies labia minora reduction. In these instances, anesthesia, antibiotic prophylaxis, and markings are performed concomitantly. My preferred technique does not necessarily follow outcome studies, because they are very limited in this field. Preoperative preparation consists of giving oral antibiotics (oral antifungal or antiviral agents are also prescribed as indicated for patients with a compatible history) the night before and the morning of surgery. Patients are instructed to shower with an antibacterial cleanser the morning of surgery. Chlorhexidine wipes are used immediately preoperatively. Usually, local anesthesia is used. These patients are instructed to apply a topical anesthetic such as LMX 5% Anorectal Cream (Ferndale Laboratories) or AneCream 5% (Focus Health Group) at least 1 hour before surgery and to cover the area with an occlusive dressing.

The planned surgical procedure is reviewed with the patient, and she is asked to change into a surgical gown. The patient should have a designated driver or postoperative caregiver; this is confirmed. Once appropriate paperwork and consent forms are obtained, the patient is given oral sedation with diazepam and alprazolam to supplement the topical anesthetics before infiltration. The cream is removed, and photos are taken with the patient in a lithotomy and a standing position, if these were not previously obtained. While the patient is standing, the superior extent of the anterior labial commissure and parts of the clitoral hood that project beyond the anterior extent of the labia majora are marked. The width of the clitoral hood, separation of the labia majora, and vertical hood redundancy are noted. The patient is placed in a lithotomy position, and markings are reinforced while assessing asymmetry of the hood and the depths of the interlabial sulcus, which may affect surgical planning or postoperative symmetry. Before the final markings are made, a pinch test is done to determine the vertical and horizontal excess. If the markings and the amount to be removed are in question, a conservative approach is recommended, but these can be confirmed intraoperatively using tailor's-tack sutures as a final check.

The relevant vulvar structures are infiltrated with either a 50:50 mixture of 1% lidocaine with 1:100,000 epinephrine and 0.5% bupivacaine with 1:100,000 epinephrine or with articaine 4% with 1:100,000 epinephrine using a 27- or 30-gauge needle. Rarely more than 2 or 3 ml of an anesthetic is required for the clitoral hood. This allows time for the epinephrine to take effect while the patient is brought to the operating suite. General anesthesia is rarely used unless requested or when combined procedures requiring it are performed.

Patient Positioning

Patients are placed in a lithotomy position and prepared in a routine sterile fashion. Satisfactory anesthesia is confirmed, and the markings are redrawn (Fig. 7-12, *A*). When a paramedian vertical reduction technique is used, either in combination with a wedge/trim labia minora reduction or as an isolated procedure, the markings (with the patient standing) at the apex of the anterior labial commissure consist of the superior limits of the dissection; this typically coincides with the hair-bearing portions of the mons pubis. Surgery above this point will result in a more visible scar and is associated with a higher incidence of inclusion cysts.

Although a variety of modalities (scalpel, scissors, electrocautery, laser, and radiofrequency) are employed for tissue resection, I use a wire- or needle-tipped electrocautery device at a low power setting, typically 8 to 12 on a ConMed electrosurgery device (Aspen ExcaliburPLUS PC) for both the Cut (Blend1) and Coag (Standard) modes. Incisions are performed using the cutting current, and the skin is resected superficial to the Buck's fascia. The cautery current is used sparingly and when needed. This essentially results in a tangential removal of skin that is commonly 2 to 3 mm in thickness; deeper dissection may result in neurovascular injury.

The following photographs demonstrate the procedure performed unilaterally. I prefer to spare a 6 to 8 mm vertical midline strip of clitoral hood skin (stretched) over the central axis of the clitoral body (Fig. 7-12, *B*). I think, but cannot prove, that this limits postoperative edema by maintaining a skin bridge and a dermal pedicle.

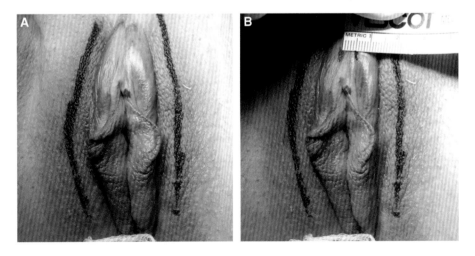

Fig. 7-12   A, This patient is prepped and draped, and the labia majora are marked. **B,** A vertical midline strip of 6 to 8 mm of clitoral hood skin (stretched) is spared over the central axis of the clitoral body.

A line is drawn medially (Fig. 7-12, *C* through *I*) and another line laterally (Fig. 7-12, *J* through *N*), preserving 6 to 8 mm of dorsal skin that inferiorly parallels the free edge of the clitoral hood by 5 to 6 mm (Fig. 7-12, *O*) as it attaches to the labia minora. The inferior extent of the clitoral hood, at its junction with the labia minora and clitoral frenulum, tends to be highly vascular and requires special attention.

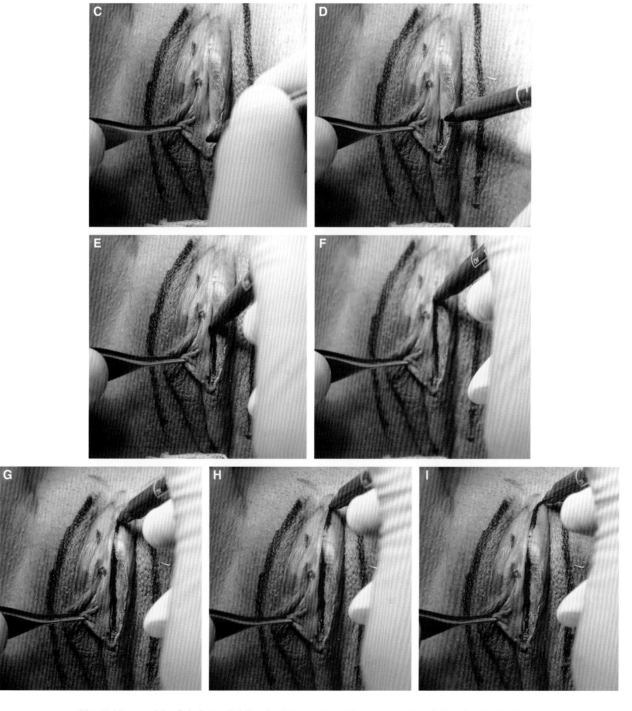

Fig. 7-12, cont'd **C-I,** A medial line is drawn preserving 6 to 8 mm of dorsal skin centrally.

Continued

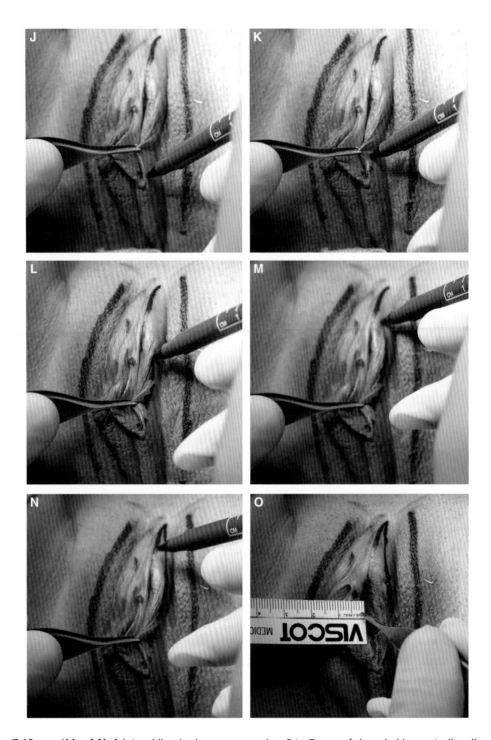

Fig. 7-12, cont'd   J-N, A lateral line is drawn preserving 6 to 8 mm of dorsal skin centrally, allowing closure to the excised intervening skin between the two lines. **O,** The medial line inferiorly parallels the free edge of the clitoral hood by 5 to 6 mm.

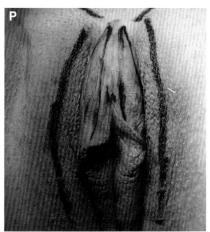 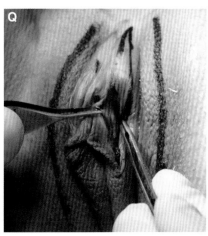 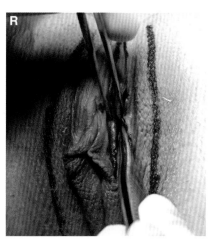

Fig. 7-12, cont'd P, Superiorly the medial line diverges to the markings made while the patient was standing. **Q** and **R,** The amount of skin to be resected (and the consequences) are determined and marked using a pinch test. Alternatively, tailor's-tack sutures can be used, if desired.

Superiorly the medial line diverges to the markings made while the patient was standing (Fig. 7-12, *P*). This demarcates the residual tissue, which will define the postoperative appearance of the clitoral hood.

The amount of skin to be resected (and the consequences) is determined and marked using a pinch test or tailor's-tack sutures, if desired (Fig. 7-12, *Q* and *R*). This will result in a second line that is lateral to the medial line.

When horizontal tissue excess is pronounced, this lateral line may rest in the interlabial sulcus. Inferiorly, the lateral markings will probably combine with the markings of the labia reduction when a combined procedure is carried out. If only a CHR is performed, the lateral markings will indicate the limits of the desired attachment of the clitoral hood with the labia minora. Superiorly, it will converge with the previously drawn paramedian line and end at the apex of the anterior labial commissure. Rarely, in patients with discernible horizontal excess, two transverse incisions in the pattern of an inverted V may be used. This will create an H-type incision. Alternatively, all incisions may converge at a single midline point to create an attenuated inverted V, but I tend to not use this design because of concerns with swelling.

Greater controversy exists over the markings along the medial edge of the labia minora. When a modified wedge is used, the medial markings consist of those for a labia minora reduction and have little to do with the clitoral hood. When combined with a trim technique and when performed as part of a composite reduction, the CHR markings are continued medial to the labia minora.

Modifications of the Medial Labia Minora Markings

There are two modifications of the medial labia minora markings. In the first approach, medial to the junction with the labia minora, the leading edge of the clitoral frenulum is excised and tapered as the incision ends before the attachment with the glans clitoris (Fig. 7-13, *A* through *D*). This is debated among surgeons but is my preferred technique.

The inset begins with estimation of the inferior extent of the attachment of the clitoral hood to the labial minora. Gentle inferior traction is employed, and the hood is sited and secured with a trifurcation suture (a half-buried horizontal mattress or two vertical mattress sutures). A similar, contralateral suture is placed, and symmetry is assessed.

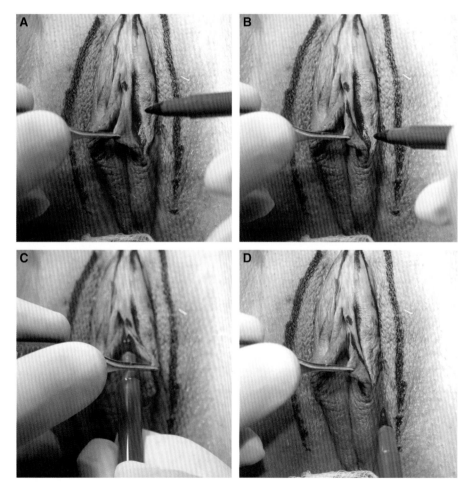

Fig. 7-13 **A-D,** Medial to the junction with the labia minora, the leading edge of the clitoral frenulum is excised and tapered as the incision ends before the attachment with the glans clitoris.

This is one of the singlemost important steps in determining the aesthetic appearance (Fig. 7-13, *E*). The clitoral frenulum is closed using a loosely running locking suture of 5-0 Vicryl Rapide buried superiorly to minimize an irritating knot in a sensitive area (Fig. 7-13, *F*). The lateral incisions are closed using a deep running suture of 5-0 Vicryl Rapide, followed by a running intracuticular suture of a 5-0 Monocryl. As a final layer, a few isolated, loose interrupted simple and vertical mattress sutures of 5-0 Vicryl Rapide are placed to finely approximate wound edges, to correct gaps and irregularities, and to reinforce the wound (Fig. 7-13, *G*). Sutures are placed loosely to accommodate the anticipated swelling and to minimize wound edge strangulation. At the conclusion of the procedure, the wound edges are infiltrated with 0.5% bupivacaine with 1:100,000 epinephrine using a 30-gauge needle for postoperative analgesia and are dressed with a bacitracin ointment–coated nonstick pad.

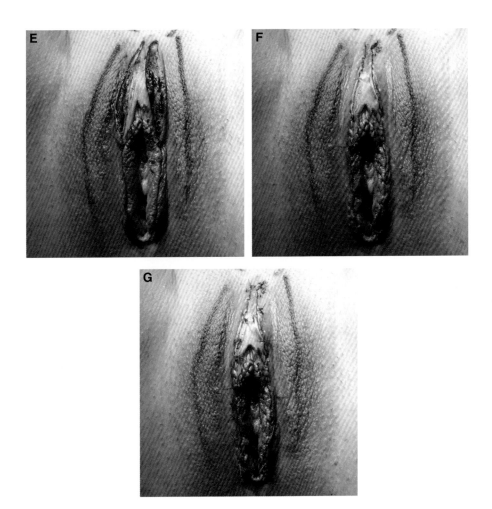

Fig. 7-13, cont'd E and **F,** The inferior extent of the clitoral hood has been inset and the clitoral frenulum closed. **G,** The repair has been reinforced with a few isolated, loose, interrupted simple and vertical mattress sutures.

In the second variation, which Gress[13] described as a treatment for clitoral protrusion, a transverse crescent of tissue leaving at least a 1.5 cm distance between the glans clitoris and the urethra is designed with a marking pen. With wound closure, the tension placed with closure of the crescent will result in a setback of the glans clitoris, whereas closure of the lateral segments will advance the clitoral hood forward, providing additional traction on the clitoral body to reduce the prominence of the clitoris.

Postoperative Care

Postoperative care is identical to that required after labia minora reduction. Patients are instructed to ice the area for the first 24 to 48 hours, as tolerated. Standard analgesic regimens are followed. Wound care consists of gentle irrigation after urination and patting after defecation. Showers are encouraged and bathing is discouraged, but sitz baths (cold is better than warm) are allowed for relief or cleansing. Patients should not use public pools, hot tubs, or saunas for 4 weeks. Limited physical activity with no exercise for 4 weeks is advised. Patients are instructed not to use tampons and to apply small amounts of ointment to sanitary pads to prevent sticking or to use nonadherent Telfa pads.

In a study measuring postoperative sensitivity after labiaplasty with CHR, transient periods of hypersensitivity of the clitoris 3 weeks after the procedure was common, similar to nipple hypersensitivity after breast augmentation.[29] Gynecologists often prescribe Dermaplast as a postoperative topical analgesic, but I have found that patients report increased relief using Neo To Go! first aid antiseptic and pain-relieving spray.

Ancillary Procedures

In a series of 407 patients undergoing labia minora and clitoral hood procedures, Alter[11] performed a clitoropexy in 35 patients (8.6%), a transverse CHR in 4 patients (1%), and a "dorsal slit of the clitoral hood" in 1 patient (0.25%). As discussed previously, Gress[13] described a modification of the CHR that corrected clitoral protrusion. Rarely, in patients with pronounced labia majora involutional atrophy, fat transfer and/or augmentation of the labia majora may provide a relative appearance of a reduced clitoral hood.

Results and Outcomes

The results of these repairs are extremely difficult to assess because of the lack of data. There are no reports on series of CHR with long-term follow-up. Because these are frequently performed in combination with labia minora reduction procedures, the complications are commonly grouped together; readers are referred to the labial reduction chapters (see Chapters 4 through 6 and 9.) As an aesthetic procedure, one of the most common complaints is persistent visibility or prominence of the clitoris and/or clitoral hood, and more aggressive resection is requested, but most practitioners advise conservative treatment.

Problems and Complications

Little has been published concerning complications, other than the outcomes discussed previously that predominantly relate to combined procedures, not those unique to the clitoral hood portion. Hamori[5] suggested that a V-Y advancement flap of the residual hood be used to provide coverage if excessive clitoral hood tissue is removed and the clitoris becomes exposed. In Alter's series[11] of 407 patients undergoing combined procedures, the only clitoral hood complications reported were one dog-ear and four suture granulomas.

According to Lean et al[23] and Minto et al,[30] surgery on the clitoris of those with ambiguous genitalia is best performed by experienced surgeons to minimize neurovascular injury, to carefully excise erectile and sensate tissue, and to achieve the best possible cosmetic result. The recurrence of clitoral phimosis after surgical release is high (greater than 50%).[31] Occasionally, irregularities of the incisions can be improved using radiofrequency resurfacing (R. Alinsod, personal communication, 2013).

References

1. Graves KL, Wilson EA, Greene JW Jr. Surgical technique for clitoral reduction. Obstet Gynecol 59:758, 1982.
2. Ostrzenski A. A new hydrodissection with reverse V-plasty technique for the buried clitoris associated with lichen sclerosis. J Gynecol Surg 26:41, 2010.
3. Tepper OM, Wulkan M, Matarasso A. Labioplasty: anatomy, etiology, and a new surgical approach. Aesthet Surg J 31:511, 2011.
4. Alter GJ. Labia minora reconstruction using clitoral hood flaps, wedge excisions, and YV advancement flaps. Plast Reconstr Surg 127:2356, 2011.
5. Hamori CA. Postoperative clitoral hood deformity after labiaplasty. Aesthet Surg J 33:1030, 2013.
6. de Alencar Felicio Y. Labial surgery. Aesthet Surg J 27:322, 2007.
7. Yavagal S, de Farias TF, Medina CA, et al. Normal vulvovaginal, perineal, and pelvic anatomy with reconstructive considerations. Semin Plast Surg 25:121, 2011.
8. Cold CJ, McGrath KA. Anatomy and histology of the penile and clitoral prepuce in primates. In Denniston GC, Hodges FM, Milos FM, eds. Male and Female Circumcision. New York: Springer, 1999.
9. van der Putte SC, Sie-Go DM. Development and structure of the glandopreputial sulcus of the human clitoris with a special reference to glandopreputial glands. Anat Rec (Hoboken) 294:156, 2011.
10. Hodgkinson DJ, Hait G. Aesthetic vaginal labioplasty. Plast Reconstr Surg 74:414, 1984.
11. Alter GJ. Aesthetic labia minora and clitoral hood reduction using extended central wedge resection. Plast Reconstr Surg 122:1780, 2008.
12. Alter GJ. Aesthetic labia minora reduction with inferior wedge resection and superior pedicle flap reconstruction. Plast Reconstr Surg 120:358, 2007.
13. Gress S. Composite reduction labiaplasty. Aesthetic Plast Surg 37:674, 2013.
14. Goodman MP. Female cosmetic genital surgery. Obstet Gynecol 113:154, 2009.
15. Hunter JG. Considerations in female external genital aesthetic surgery techniques. Aesthet Surg J 28:106, 2008.
16. Hamori CA. Aesthetic surgery of the female genitalia: labiaplasty and beyond. Plast Reconstr Surg 134:661, 2014.

17. Ostrzenski A. Clitoral subdermal hoodoplasty for medical indications and aesthetic motives. A new technique. J Reprod Med 58:149, 2012.
18. Benson R. Clitoral hood reduction. Presented at the Seventh Annual Congress for Aesthetic Vaginal Surgery, Tucson, AZ, Jan 2012.
19. Lloyd J, Crouch NS, Minto CL, et al. Female genital appearance: "normality" unfolds. BJOG 112:643, 2005.
20. Ostrzenski A. Selecting aesthetic gynecologic procedures for plastic surgeons: a review of target methodology. Aesthetic Plast Surg 37:256, 2013.
21. Shaw D, Lefebvre G, Bouchard C, et al; Society of Obstetricians and Gynaecologists of Canada. Female genital cosmetic surgery. J Obstet Gynaecol Can 35:1108, 2013.
22. Foldès P, Droupy S, Cuzin B. [Cosmetic surgery of the female genitalia] Prog Urol 23:601, 2013.
23. Lean WL, Hutson JM, Deshpande AV, et al. Clitoroplasty: past, present and future. Pediatr Surg Int 23:289, 2007.
24. Alter GJ. Central wedge nymphectomy with a 90-degree Z-plasty for aesthetic reduction of the labia minora. Plast Reconstr Surg 115:2144, 2005.
25. Alter GJ. A new technique for aesthetic labia minora reduction. Ann Plast Surg 40:287, 1998.
26. Gress S. [Aesthetic and functional corrections of the female genital area] Gynakol Geburtshilfliche Rundsch 47:23, 2006.
27. Apesos J, Jackson R, Miklos JR, et al, eds. Vagina Makeover & Rejuvenation. Cape Town: MWP Media, 2008.
28. Triana L, Robledo AM. Aesthetic surgery of female external genitalia. Aesthet Surg J 35:165, 2015.
29. Placik OJ, Arkins JA. A prospective evaluation of female external genitalia sensitivity to pressure following labia minora reduction and clitoral hood reduction. Plast Reconstr Surg 136:442e, 2015.
30. Minto CL, Liao LM, Woodhouse CR, et al. The effect of clitoral surgery on sexual outcome in individuals who have intersex conditions with ambiguous genitalia: a cross-sectional study. Lancet 361:1252, 2003.
31. Smith YR, Haefner HK. Vulvar lichen sclerosis. Am J Clin Dermatol 5:105, 2004.

CHAPTER 8

Augmentation of the Labia Majora With Fat Grafting

Lina Triana, Paul E. Banwell

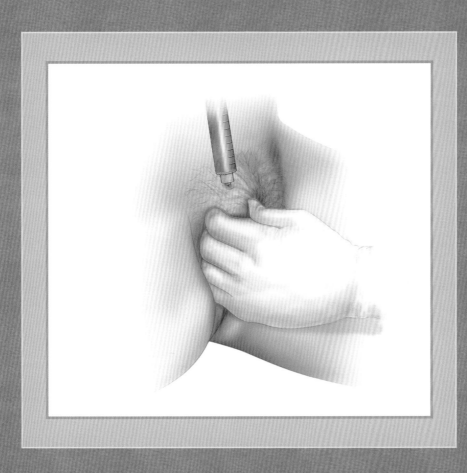

Key Points

- *The main indications for augmentation of the labia majora are hypoplasia, loose skin, or both.*

- *If the labia majora are very "baggy" with significant excess skin, then excisional labia majora reduction should also be considered. Treatment options include autologous fat grafting and the use of dermal fillers.*

- *When performing only fat grafting in patients with a lot of loose skin, surgeons should not place too much fat in the inferior third of the labia majora. Patients who desire a lot of fullness should be informed that more than one procedure needs to be performed.*

Why Perform Augmentation of the Labia Majora?

The aim of this chapter is to describe a nonsurgical approach to labia majora augmentation with autologous fat transfer. This procedure may be performed alone or in conjunction with other aesthetic external genital surgical procedures to enhance results.

In today's society we are more aware of genital appearance because of the current vogue for the minimal pubic hair appearance and the increased discussion in the media and popular press.[1]

In particular, smooth and prominent labia majora may provide a more youthful appearance to the female genitalia. Women today mostly seem to desire the youthful appearance of concealed labia minora and full, smooth labia majora.

Techniques that return fullness to the labia majora are therefore important in cosmetic surgeons' armamentarium for addressing the external genital. Autologous fat transfer, through lipomodeling, is a well-described technique to enhance the appearance of the labia majora and an important procedure in vulvar plastic surgery.[2,3]

Indications and Contraindications

The main indications for augmentation of the labia majora are hypoplasia, loose skin, or both.

Labia majora hypoplasia and/or laxity has several causes, and these may be classified as congenital or acquired. Acquired causes include changes secondary to trauma or tumors but also physiologic causes such as aging and those associated with menopause or changes during pregnancy. Massive-weight-loss patients may also present with significant bagginess and loss of volume.

Many younger patients with otherwise seemingly "normal" labia majora may desire only puffier, fuller labia majora, because this may be perceived as an aesthetic ideal.

There are no significant contraindications for augmentation to this area. Surgeons must warn patients of potential infection, but this risk is no greater than with any other female genital surgery. In very thin patients with minimal fat deposition, lack of a good donor area may be considered a relative contraindication, and surgical planning and discussion with the patient is paramount in these circumstances.

Anatomy

The anatomy of the female external genitalia has been described in Chapter 1.

Embryologically, the labia majora in women are derived from the genital swellings that, in the male fetus, develop into the scrotum.[1] They are two cutaneous specialized skin folds that extend posteriorly from the mons pubis; they become wider than the labia minora anteriorly and start to narrow posteriorly.[3] They enclose the internal structures of the female genitalia, especially in nulliparous women, although the anatomic appearance may vary widely.

The labia majora have a hairy outer face and an inner face that lacks hair and has a finer skin for cutaneous annexes and semimucosal glandular cover. The labia majora are naturally filled with subcutaneous fatty tissue to varying degrees.

The blood supply to the labia majora is from the posterior labial artery and the perineal artery, both branches of the internal pudendal artery. The nerve supply arises from the pudendal nerve.

Clinical Evaluation and Planning

Cosmetic genital surgery is no different from the rest of our aesthetic plastic surgery practice; thus listening to patients is of paramount importance. The motivation for presentation should be discussed in detail, including perceived expectations and understanding of the complications.

The examination is then performed. We recommend patients use of a mirror while in the lithotomy and standing positions so that their concerns can be pointed out and conveyed effectively. Careful documentation of the anatomy, including any variations, should be encouraged for medicolegal purposes.

If the labia majora are very "baggy" with significant excess skin, then excisional labia majora reduction should also be considered (see Chapter 6). The discussion and decisions about the degree of filling with fat should be similar to those involving breast implant sizing. The decisions should be made after listening carefully to the patient to understand the end result she desires. We must always inform patients that some amount of fat will be resorbed after labia majora lipomodeling.

Surgical Technique

The Coleman fat transfer technique has been well described.[4] Surgeons often have their own personalized technique for harvesting, preparing, and injecting fat according to available equipment and personal preference. The procedure can be performed with the patient under local anesthesia in an office setting, depending on local regulations in each country. No blocks are needed.

Markings

If fat grafting alone is performed, then we recommend marking the area with the patient in the lithotomy position. A long, oval-shaped outline is drawn, starting at the level of the outer introitus and extending to the level of the pubic prominence (2 to 3 cm above the distal upper part of the clitoral hood).

Harvesting the Fat Graft

The fat graft can be taken from an area where it is available in excess. Areas such as the inner thighs and inner knees are easily accessed, because they are in the proximity of the area to be filled.

The area to be liposuctioned for obtaining the fat graft is also marked, and tumescent solution may be injected in the subcutaneous tissue, according to normal practice. Our tumescent solution is prepared using 500 ml saline solution, 1 adrenaline ampule (1:1000), and 25 ml 1% lidocaine (Fig. 8-1).

Usually, about 80 to 120 cc of fat may be obtained by liposuction using 10 ml syringes or approximately three times as much fat as planned for use in the fat graft. We prefer to use a 1.8 to 2.0 mm cannula for extracting fat. This same cannula can be used to apply the tumescent solution if required.

Several techniques have been described to harvest and process the fat such as centrifuging, washing and straining, and decantation (Fig. 8-2).

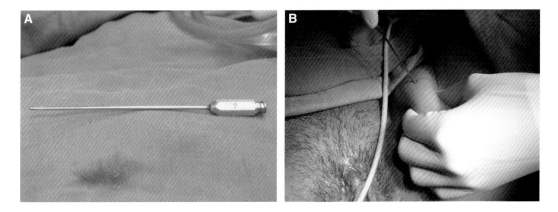

Fig. 8-1 A, Cannula used for fat harvest. **B,** The most common site of fat extraction is the inner thighs.

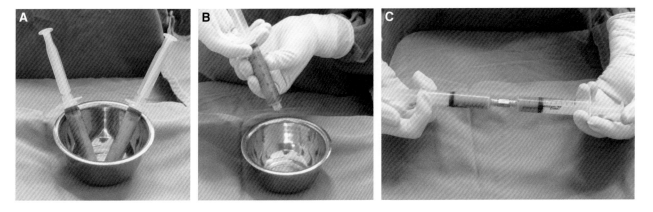

Fig. 8-2 Autologous fat graft preparation. **A,** Fat decantation. **B,** Elimination of liquid, preserving fat. **C,** Fat transfer from one syringe to another to obtain a thinner consistency.

In 1994 Coleman[4-7] devised a protocol in fat grafting, for which he coined the name *LipoStructure.* This innovative protocol minimized the traumatic maneuvers with adipose tissue and optimized the viability of the injected fat cells. Other authors have since described different techniques in fat harvesting and preparation. Analysis of adipocyte morphology suggests that the number of altered cells is statistically higher in centrifuged specimens than in sedimented specimens.[8]

We prefer to harvest fat with regular 10 ml syringes and cannulas and to process samples using simple decantation.

Injecting Fat Into the Labia Majora

The patient is placed in the lithotomy position on the operating room table.

Incisions are placed, one on each side above the labia majora. Placement of these incisions is crucial to ensure the whole length of the labia is treated. Placing these too low sometimes leads to deficiencies in superior aspect fill. Fig. 8-3 shows examples of injection and molding.

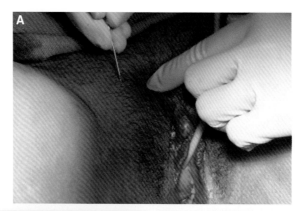

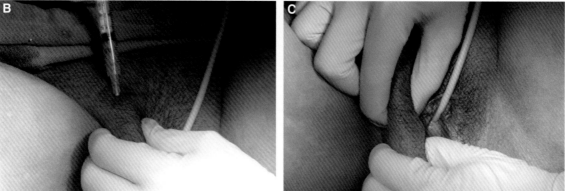

Fig. 8-3   Lipoinjection of autologous fat graft. **A,** Insertion of the syringe where we want the fat to stay. **B,** Autologous fat graft injection. **C,** Molding of the fat.

Excellent injection technique is crucial to prevent fat lakes, which can occur with necrosis and/or cyst formation. A layered, "spaghetti"-type approach with injections into the deep and superficial layers is essential to prevent these issues.

When fat is introduced, one hand is placed on the syringe itself and softly pushes the syringe embolus, while the other hand is in the marked area guiding the fat to where it needs to stay as it is actively introduced.

Fat is injected evenly into the labia majora until the desired size is achieved (Fig. 8-4). At the end of the procedure, the surgeon molds the fat with both hands.

Postoperative Care

Swelling and tenderness are expected for up to 4 weeks. No special recommendations are given to patients other than to avoid strenuous exercise and sexual intercourse for 4 weeks.

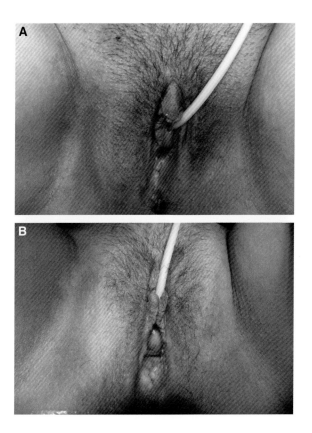

Fig. 8-4 Fat grafting lipoinjection. **A,** Lipoinjection on the right side. **B,** Bilateral lipoinjection.

Results and Outcomes

The objective with labia majora augmentation is to produce labia that are fuller and more youthful. The use of fat injections may achieve this desired outcome,[9] but integration of the fat graft is variable, and some patients require secondary procedures to satisfy their expectations[8] (Figs. 8-5 through 8-7).

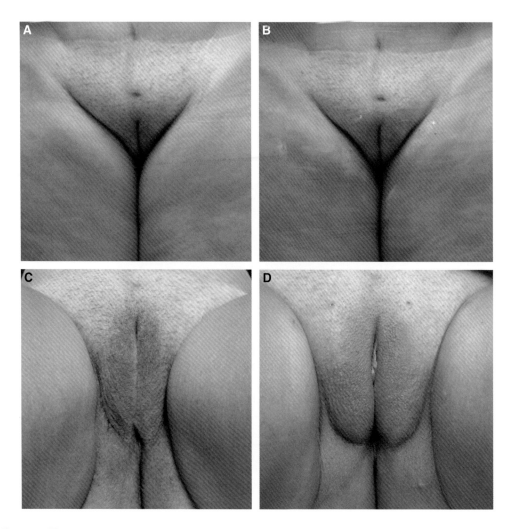

Fig. 8-5   This 57-year-old woman underwent labiaplasty with lipomodeling. **A** and **C,** Preoperative appearance. **B** and **D,** Postoperative result.

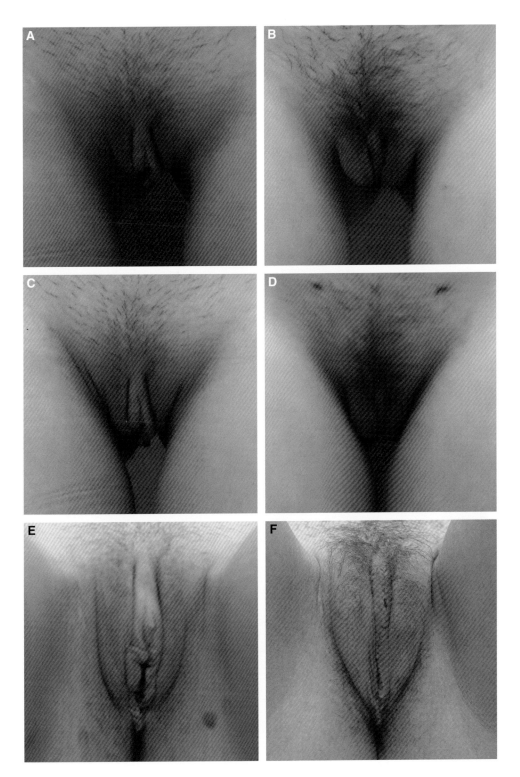

Fig. 8-6 This 32-year-old woman had resection of the labia minora and lipomodeling of the labia majora in the same procedure. **A, C,** and **E,** Preoperative appearance. **B, D,** and **F,** Postoperative results.

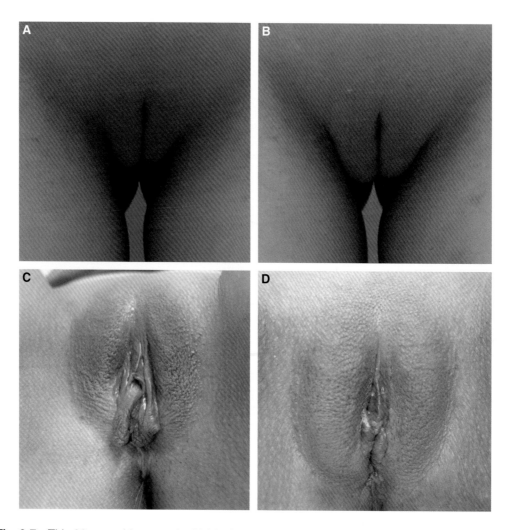

Fig. 8-7 This 32-year-old woman had labiaplasty and lipomodeling. **A** and **C**, Preoperative appearance. **B** and **D**, Postoperative results.

Problems and Complications

During the whole fat grafting procedure, we must consider that we want the labia majora to have a thinner appearance inferiorly and a wider appearance of the superior aspect. If only fat grafting is performed on a patient with a lot of loose skin, excessive fat must not be placed in the inferior third of the labia majora. This mistake is easily made, because usually this area has a larger amount of loose skin.

Fat injections are technically less complicated than other augmentation procedures and leave smaller scars, but fat reabsorption can be variable in the labia majora and, in some cases, unpredictable. Patients should be counseled about this before surgery. Those who desire a lot of fullness should be informed that more than one procedure needs to be performed. In such situations, staged procedures should be scheduled a minimum of 3 months apart to encourage optimal vascular conditions for further graft take.

Fat cysts can be expected in as many of 30% of cases. Most are not visible and only palpable to the patient. We advise telling patients to routinely massage them to help decrease their size and improve hypersensitivity.

Fat necrosis can occur and may result in fat infection if not treated expediently. If fat necrosis is suspected, extraction of liquefied fat through extra incisions may be warranted. Fat necrosis may present as an area of inflammation and/or soreness and usually decreases after oral antibiotics are given. However, drainage of the fat is always advisable if symptoms persist.

Conclusion

Labia majora augmentation using autologous fat transfer may improve the appearance of the vaginal and perineal areas without visible scars while preserving normal sensitivity to the region.[10] This technique is an important part of our armamentarium in aesthetic surgery of the female genitalia, in association with other procedures.

References

1. Hamori CA. Aesthetic surgery of the female genitalia: labiaplasty and beyond. Plast Reconstr Surg 134:661, 2014.
2. Mirzabeigi MN, Jandali S, Mettel RK, et al. The nomenclature of "vaginal rejuvenation" and elective vulvovaginal plastic surgery. Aesthet Surg J 31:723, 2011.
3. Triana L, Robledo AM. Aesthetic surgery of female external genitalia. Aesthet Surg J 35:165, 2015.
4. Coleman SR. Structural fat grafts: the ideal filler? Clin Plast Surg 28:111, 2001.
5. Coleman SR. Hand rejuvenation with structural fat grafting. Plast Reconstr Surg 110:1731, 2002.
6. Coleman SR. Long-term survival of fat transplants: controlled demonstrations. Aesthetic Plast Surg 19:421, 1995.
7. Coleman SR. Facial recontouring with lipostructure. Clin Plast Surg 24:347, 1997.
8. Lin JY, Wang C, Pu LL. Can we standardize the techniques for fat grafting? Clin Plast Surg 42:199, 2015.
9. Triana L, Robledo AM. Refreshing labioplasty techniques for plastic surgeons. Aesthetic Plast Surg 36:1078, 2012.
10. Vogt PM, Herold C, Rennekampff HO. Autologous fat transplantation for labia majora reconstruction. Aesthetic Plast Surg 35:913, 2011.

CHAPTER 9

Augmentation of the Labia Majora With Fillers

Nicolas Berreni

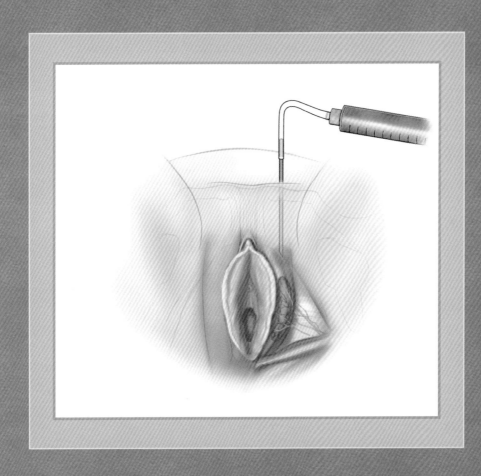

Key Points

- *The use of specific injectable hyaluronic acids (HAs) for the reconstruction and remodeling of the labia majora provides an effective, reversible, and safe treatment that is dependent on surgeons' excellent anatomic and functional knowledge of the genital area, their mastery of the technique, and the quality of the products used.*

- *Rejuvenation or restoration of the vulvovaginal region with heterogeneous biodegradable products such as HA promises to be an area of extensive development, especially in synergy with other current or future nonsurgical methods.*

The labia majora play a vital role in protecting the labia minora (nymphs) in the superior part of the vestibule and the introitus (lower third of the vagina) in the posterior part. This protection prevents unwanted friction of the labia minora, particularly friction pain from sports activities (for example, horseback riding and bicycling) or tight and form-fitting clothes. Hypotrophy of the labia majora is a cause of chronic vulvitis and vulvovaginal dryness, causing discomfort, pruritus, and intromission dyspareunia. Functional, psychological, and sexual consequences are real limitations in women's lives and can affect sexuality, libido, and self-confidence.

The aesthetic of the vulval area depends on the blending of the mons pubis subcutaneous tissues covering the pubic bone with the upper labia majora.

The growing desire of women to correct or retain the youthful appearance of a more sensual genital area was probably amplified by the growing popularity of pubic and vulval hair removal,[1] but it also results from the desire to erase the consequences of aging, childbirth, and various injuries. Anatomic understanding of the vulvovaginal region is essential to the practice of genital rejuvenation and restoration techniques. The intricate complexity of the relationship between the superficial and deep structures and the intimate relationships among the skin, mucous membranes, muscles, ligaments, and fascia define these anatomic and functional units.[2]

Anatomy and Histology

The labia majora are formed by a skin surface comprising stratified squamous epithelium (keratinized and pigmented), dense vascular dermis rich in sebaceous glands, apocrine

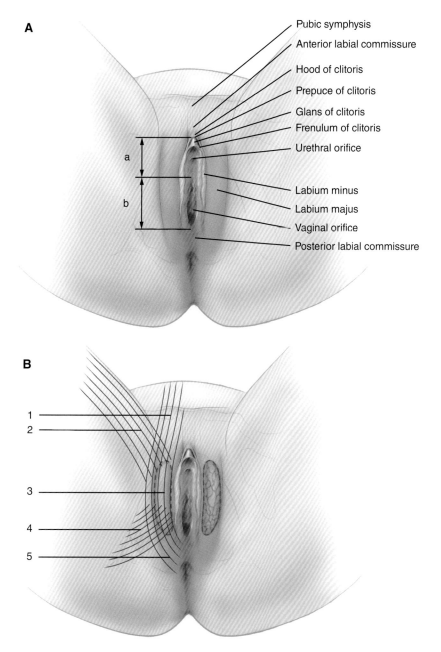

Fig. 9-1 A, The superficial perineum. **B,** Dissection of the corpus under the dermis and superficial fat to view the labial fat. (*a,* Urethral part of vestibule; *b,* hymenal part of vestibule; *1,* puboclitoris conjunctive expansion; *2,* inguinal expansion; *3,* labial adipose corpus; *4,* gluteal expansion; *5,* perineal expansion.)

glands, and a deep layer of smooth muscle fibers: the labial dartos (Fig. 9-1). Other components of the labia majora include a fatty layer under the skin that regresses with aging or excessive weight loss and a labial fat corpus, which is both a fibrofatty formation rich in vessels and a semierectile organ reinforced by elastic fibers with fibrous expansions that push it forward, sideways, and backward. Regression of fatty tissue of the labia results from the gravitational effect of body weight on the perineum and from the repetitive friction movement of the thighs.

During aging, the skin surface of the labia undergoes the same degradation as the body's dermis. The labia majora fatty subcutaneous plane undergoes a "fat melting" or lipoatrophy. This creates a deflated appearance and hypotonicity, with volume loss of the filling material and a wrinkled appearance of the skin surface. This loss of protection also affects the labia minora and vestibule, which results in vulvovaginal dryness, spontaneous or induced pain during sexual intercourse, and compensatory hypertrophy of the labia minora by sliding of the dermis.[3] Hypotonia associated with subcutaneous lipoatrophy causes the dermis overlying the labia majora to relax and extend into the dermis of the outer face of the labia minora, increasing their relief.

The main principles of the remodeling or restoration of the labia majora are based on reconstruction of the different planes:

- Superficial labia majora dermal rejuvenation is similar to the rejuvenation and biorevitalization of the dermis of the face:
    - Non-cross-linked or weakly cross-linked HA injected intradermally or superficially by needle, roller, microneedle, or injector gun according to well-known techniques in mesotherapy
    - The use of platelet-rich plasma in multiple injections, alone or combined with HA, which allows a remarkable reconstruction of the thickness of the dermis, eliminating vulval wrinkles, fine lines, and folds.
- Deep dermal labia majora rejuvenation treatments improve the tone of the labial and vulval muscles (dartos), the trophicity, and the youthful appearance of the labia majora. Radiofrequency techniques and thermal effects applied to the genital area remarkably correct vulvovaginal loss from aging or trauma of childbirth through its effects on neocollagenesis and smooth muscle tone (see Chapter 16).
- In continuity with the fatty tissue of the pubic region, the fatty tissue of the labia helps to enhance the relief of the labia majora and distinguish between the hairy external side and the glabrous inner side. This subcutaneous fat is made up of a superficial layer and a deep level that covers the surface area of the perineum. The Bartholin glands and erectile bodies, with their various muscles and fascias, are located between the superficial fascia of the perineum and the perineal membrane (or the lower fascia of the urogenital diaphragm), which comes in contact with the deep layers of fatty tissue. Bulbospongiosus muscles cover the vestibular bulbs, and ischiocavernosus muscles overlie the corpora cavernosa[3] (Fig. 9-2).

The loss of thickness of the fatty tissue associated with causes such as aging (after menopause), estrogen loss, significant weight loss (postpartum weight loss), and everyday microtrauma (from sports, tight clothes, hair removal) can accelerate skin aging. This results in a general "loosening" with collapse of the vulval relief skin and deep wrinkles. The outline of the labia majora—with an outer surface, an inner surface, and a protruding free edge—is created by the same subcutaneous fatty tissue. It gives the appearance of an inverted V.

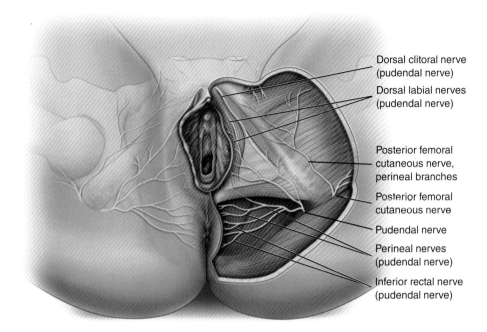

Dorsal clitoral nerve
(pudendal nerve)

Dorsal labial nerves
(pudendal nerve)

Posterior femoral
cutaneous nerve,
perineal branches

Posterior femoral
cutaneous nerve

Pudendal nerve

Perineal nerves
(pudendal nerve)

Inferior rectal nerve
(pudendal nerve)

Fig. 9-2   The superficial perineal fascia and perineal membrane.

Correcting this fatty atrophy by injections of HA is an alternative to lipofilling. This nonsurgical, minimally invasive genital rejuvenation method is particularly attractive for its simplicity of implementation, its in-office practice facility, and its convincing results.

Indications and Contraindications

Indications

- Women older than 18 years of age
- Patients who desire aesthetic rejuvenation of the labia majora or to protect the vulva and the labia minora

Contraindications

- Male sex
- Pregnant or breast-feeding women
- Known hypersensitivity to one of the injected components (for example, HA and mannitol)
- Vulvovaginal infections in the injection site (bacterial, viral such as herpes or HPV, or fungal)
- Skin problems like inflammation near the injection area
- The presence of semipermanent or permanent products in the area to be treated
- Recent vulval surgery in the treatment area or progressive recent or nearby cancers

Contraindications Related to Hyaluronic Acid

- A history of autoimmune disease, streptococcus disease, or acute rheumatic fever with cardiac localization

Patient Evaluation

The assessment of lipoatrophic labia majora, and therefore the amount needed to be injected, is made by comparing and assessing the thickness of the pubic fat and the protrusion of the labia minora. We need to find an aesthetic and functional balance between these structures.

Preoperative Planning and Preparation

Patients are given 3 days' antiseptic treatment with intravaginal ovules of neomycin with polymyxin B and nystatin. During the 3 days before the intervention, no hair is removed from the vulva by shaving or any other means.

We ask patients with significant vulval hair growth to perform a "deburring" 2 or 3 days before the procedure. This involves cutting the hair with scissors to a length of 1 cm.

Before the injection, a careful surgical antiseptic prep is performed, with at least three passes throughout the dermal surface, the vulva, and intravaginally. (We usually use povidone iodine 10%, occasionally, chlorhexidine gluconate or benzalkonium chloride.)

Surgical Technique

Anesthesia

Xylocaine 2% is injected intradermally, 0.2 ml on each side. These injection sites will be used again. We also inject deeply and subcutaneously (five to seven injections of 0.3 ml) along the future path of the cannula, following the line previously drawn, described below.

Markings

Several points of introduction are possible, depending on the position and preference of the operator. Fig. 9-3 shows points that are safer and more consistent with anatomic characteristics. The upper points I use are in the lateropubic area, two to three finger-breadths on each side of a vertical center line, between the pubis and the posterior commissure. The lower points and the points 2 cm lateral to the labia minora constitute the

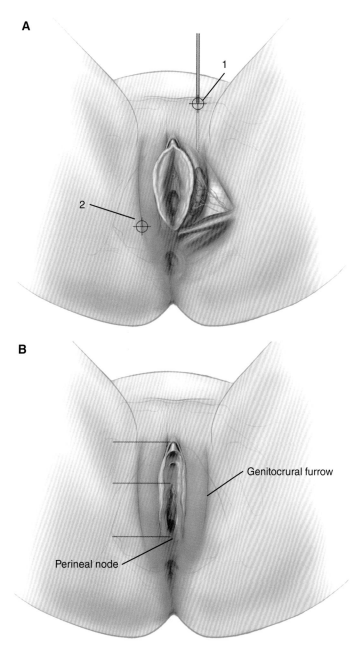

Fig. 9-3 Location of points of possible injection. **A,** Upper points (*1* and *2*). The injection plan must stay in the superficial fat under the skin, well above the deep fat and the bulbospongiosus muscle. **B,** Lower point.

posterior commissure. For these injections, the patient is in a lithotomy position, and the surgeon inserts the needle or the injection cannula upward and diagonally toward the genitocrural furrow.

Dotted lines are drawn on the skin along the proposed cannula pathway. The direction should be oblique, oriented toward the perineal node without overflowing inside the free edge of the labia and the external remote genitocrural furrow. We stop below the posterior commissure and just above the perineal center.

Patient Positioning

The patient can be placed either in a gynecologic position with the legs slightly parted or supine on a simple clinical examination table (Fig. 9-4). The practitioner can be positioned as when performing a pelvic examination, sitting on a stool. (An electric, adjustable table is essential for optimal visibility and working comfort.) When performing lipofilling, I prefer to stand on the same side I am injecting.

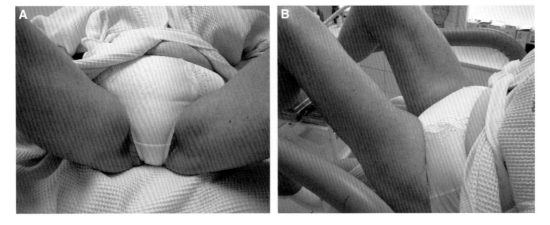

Fig. 9-4 A, The practitioner may be seated in front of the patient, who is positioned as for a gynecologic examination. **B,** A more favorable position is to stand on the side of the patient, who is supine on the table.

Technique

Materials

The following supplies are needed for this procedure (Fig. 9-5):

- Needles: Length 13 mm, 20 mm, 25 mm; diameter 27-gauge to 30-gauge
- Cannulas: Length 80 mm; diameter 18-gauge
- Xylocaine 2%
- Compresses, gloves
- Syringes of HA: 2 ml per syringe
- Pens and/or markers

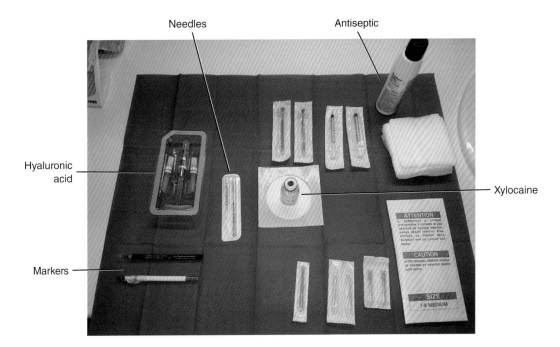

Fig. 9-5   Supplies needed for the procedure.

Hyaluronic Acid

HA is a high-molecular-weight anionic polymer. It is a member of the nonsulfated glycosaminoglycan superfamily, and its structure is based on the linear repetition of disaccharide sequences (D-glucuronic acid and D-N-acetylglucosamine).

HA is endogenously synthesized. It is naturally present in many tissues and plays important physiologic roles in living organisms, including maintenance of the viscoelasicity of liquid connective tissues such as synovial fluid in the joints and eye vitreous humor; control of tissue hydration, especially in the dermis, mucous membranes, and submucosal tissue layers; water transport; proteoglycan organization in the extracellular matrix; tissue repair; and various receptor-mediated functions in cell detachment, tumor management, and inflammation.[4] One of the most important features of this molecule is its conservation across species. HA structure appears identical throughout phyla and species as diverse as *Pseudomonas* slime, *Ascaris* worms and mammals such as the rat, rabbit, and humans.[5]

Endogenous HA turnover is controlled by HA synthases (isoforms 1, 2, and 3) and hyaluronidases (Hyal-1, Hyal-2, and Hyal-3) and appears to be relatively fast: The normal HA half-life ranges from 3 weeks in the cartilage to 2 days in the dermis.[6] This aspect of HA metabolism was critical in the early 1990s, when injectable HA-based products were released on the market. The fast endogenous turnover necessitated transforming and strengthening the HA-based gels to prolong their clinical effects. Thus the solution was found in the cross-linking process. Basically, it is a simple reaction between a chemical and HA fibers. The goal is to create covalent, stable chemical bonds to bring HA fibers closer. By performing this step, hyaluronidase accessibility to the HA network decreases drastically. The created covalent bonds will affect the rheology of the product, especially viscosity and elasticity parameters. To date, available products on the market are cross-linked with diepoxyoctane, polyethyleneglycol, or 1,4-butanediol diglycidylether.

In gynecology, HA was first studied because of its demonstrated postoperative antiadhesion properties.[7] It was also widely used as an important ingredient in topical hydrating and lubricating gels or injected for conditions such as dyspareunia.[8] Because of the increasing interest in HA-based fillers for facial volumizing in plastic surgery, using this product as a new tool to treat age-related fat lysis of the female genitalia seemed logical. More specifically, labia majora atrophy seemed to be the perfect target to begin those treatments. A lot of papers have been published to describe labia majora fat grafting techniques.[9-11] These procedures are performed in an operating room, and an initial overcorrection is often needed because of the classical postoperative grafted fat resorption. To easily compensate for this loss, HA-based gels were developed.

Labia majora fat injections with HA should be adapted to this anatomic layer. Subcutaneous fat is present in the superficial, middle, and deep skin layers of the labia majora (Fig. 9-6). The HA injection plan must be adapted to the specific anatomic location. Many products on the facial market are designed to be injected in the fat, but can labia

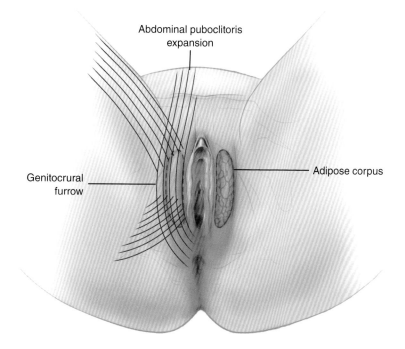

Abdominal puboclitoris
expansion

Genitocrural
furrow

Adipose corpus

Fig. 9-6 The adipose corpus and extensions of different connected fascias.

majora fat be considered as equivalent to facial fat? The genotypic profile of labia majora adipocytes has not been specifically studied yet, but anatomically, labia majora fat is connected to superficial Camper fascia, and also to deeper Colles fascia (which is comparable to Scarpa fascia in labia majora). Colles fascia is the extension of the superficial fascia of the abdominal wall. It is attached to the ischiopubic muscular rami and to the urogenital diaphragm; thus this fat compartment is subject to high mechanical constraints: The mechanical stresses on the labia are related to pressure forces created by gravity, body weight, friction of the thighs, extensive walking, sports activities, and the pressure transmitted by abdominal contraction on the perineum.

Moreover, the labia majora are anatomic structures primarily dedicated to protection and shock absorption. For all these reasons, labia majora fat is different from facial fat. Thus injected HA gel characteristics should be adapted to this specific environment to prevent product migration after the treatment.

Because of the anatomic, functional, and sexual importance of the genital area, particularly the labia majora, we need to choose the products we use carefully. Many injectable HAs have been created as "volumizing" fillers, including Voluma (Allergan), which is commonly used for this indication, Belotero (Merz), Sculptra (Sanofi), and Radiesse (Bioform Medical). But these FDA-approved products are intended for facial rejuvenation. Although good results can be achieved using these products in the genital area, they are off label for this use. The product technical adaptation for the indication and legal and safety concerns should never be disregarded. Only one product (Desirial Plus, Vivacy) has been clinically tested and received European approval for this very specific indication. It is not FDA approved yet. This product also contains mannitol, a natural component of plant origin that can delay the degradation of hyaluronic acid by the native hyaluronidase and free radicals produced during injection.

Desirial Plus is the product I use specifically for vulval remodeling. It has undergone several clinical studies. The final product is the result of a "compromise" between different physicochemical characteristics that characterize HAs, including viscosity, molecular weight, concentration (21 mg/g), single-phase specificity, elasticity, fluidity, cross-linking, hygroscopicity. Thus the volumizing-type product may be perfectly suited for genital applications and previously mentioned constraints.

Because the rheologic behavior of HA-based fillers is very different from that of grafted fat, the injected volume should not be compared directly. In 2011 Vogt et al[11] published a case report in which 52 ml of fat was injected to correct labia majora asymmetry. This volume is not achievable with HA-based fillers. However, with 1 to 4 ml of HA, good and natural-appearing corrections are possible because of the high elasticity level of gels compared with that of grafted fat. HA-based fillers can also be used for touch-up procedures after fat grafting surgery.

Method

After xylocaine 2% is injected, we wait a few minutes for it to take effect. We make a small hole using a 27-gauge needle and introduce a cannula of 8 cm with an 18-gauge diameter. The entire cannula is introduced following the marked line and is advanced strictly subcutaneously. HA is injected in a retrograde fashion from bottom to top (Fig. 9-7).

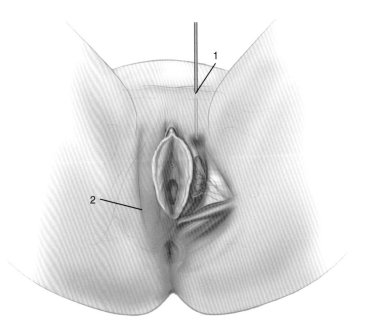

Fig. 9-7 Cannula introduction from an upper point.

The advantages of this injection method are that it allows perfect visualization and harmonious product distribution as the injection is controlled between the thumb and index finger. We try to create a feminine appearance and youthful, "sensual" labia!

After the injections, we digitally massage the area for a homogeneous distribution of the product and harmonious aesthetic results.

Postoperative Care

Patients are instructed not to participate in sexual activities, bathing, swimming, and sports. They should not wear tight underwear for 1 week.

Results and Outcomes

This 25-year-old woman was concerned with the wrinkled appearance of her vulva and the serious repercussions on her sex life (Fig. 9-8). I injected 2 ml of HA (Desirial Plus) in each labium majus.

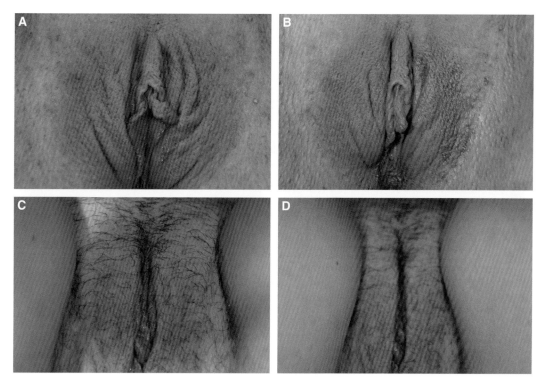

Fig. 9-8 A, This patient, a professional kite surfer, is shown before the injections. **B,** Immediately after the injections. **C,** One month after the injections. **D,** Three months after the injections.

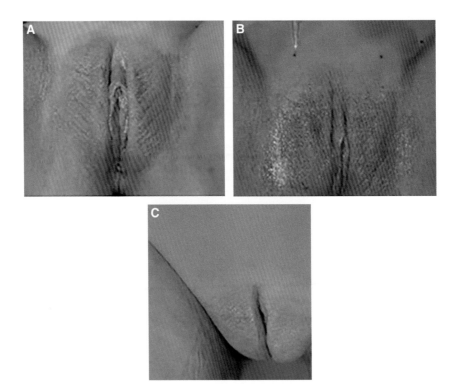

Fig. 9-9   A, The patient is shown before the injections. **B,** During the injections. **C,** Six months after the injections.

This 45-year-old woman underwent progestin therapy for 10 years for gynecologic pathology. The therapy had serious effects on her vulval dermis and caused labial lipoatrophy. I injected 2 ml of HA (Desirial Plus) in each labium majus (Fig. 9-9).

Fig. 9-10 shows how Desirial Plus injections resulted very significant improvement of functional disorders, as reported by patients.

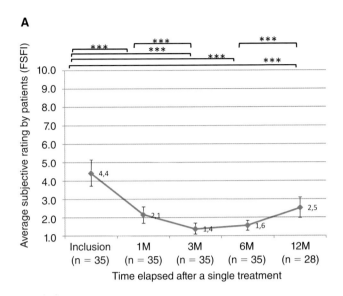

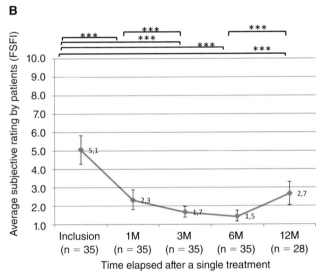

Fig. 9-10 Confirmation of a very significant average reduction of itching and vulvar chafing in a population of 35 patients and a high durability of effect (longer than 6 months) after a single treatment with Desirial Plus. **A,** Itching. **B,** Chafing. (*FSFI,* Female Sexual Function Index.)

Problems and Complications

Complications related to lipofilling of the labia are reported in Chapter 8. Unlike surgical techniques such as those using autologous fat injections (lipofilling) for reshaping the labia majora, complications of HA injections are very rare and often related to technical problems. Complications of Desirial Plus injections in the labia are associated with poor injection technique and distribution of filler. These include creating nodules of heterogeneous clusters and unsightly labial relief, including a "pudding" appearance, columns, or "testicles."

Injections into the labial adipose corpus can cause hematomas, cysts, painful lymphangitis, or dysharmonious distribution of the filler product that creates a nodular appearance. The result has been described as "socks," or "pillars."

Theoretically, as with facial HA injections, a nodule or granuloma may result from inflammatory hyperimmune reactivity, which will require specific treatment (corticosteroids) or excision.

Physicians need to respect the specific conditions of injection techniques and mark the safety zones around the labia majora. Most problems are minor and easy to resolve (Table 9-1). Leakage and the total loss of the product injected into the ischiorectal fat have occurred (Fig. 9-11).

Table 9-1 *Known Negative Effects of Desirial Plus Treatment**	
Side Effect	Percentage of Patients Affected
Ecchymosis (light to moderate)	3
Pain during injection (light to moderate)	6
Transient edema (light to moderate)	9
Pain during postinjection massages (light to moderate)	6
Redness/erythema (light to moderate)	9

*There are also classic and transitional effects that do not last long.
The results of the clinical study of more than 50 patients confirmed that the negative effects occur in less than 10% of cases and are identical to those of any injection.

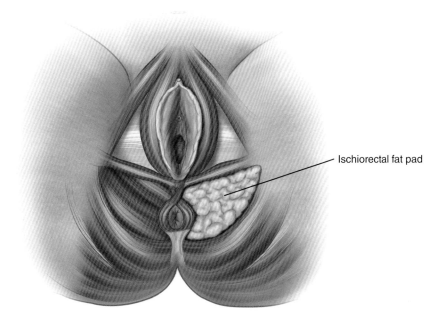

Fig. 9-11   Continuity between the labial fat and ischiorectal fat.

References

1. Herbenick D, Schick V, Reece M, et al. Pubic hair removal among women in the United States: prevalence, methods and characteristics. J Sex Med 7:3322, 2010.
2. Nicolas Berreni. The aesthetic gynecology, an innovation. Université Nice Sophia Antipolis, 2013.
3. Kamina P. Anatomie clinique de l'appareil génital féminin. Encyclopedia Gynecological Surgical Medicine, 1993.
4. Kogan G, Soltes L, Stern R, et al. Hyaluronic acid: its function degradation in in vivo systems. In Atta-ur-Rahmanm, ed. Studies in Natural Product Chemistry, vol 34. Philadelphia: Elsevier Science, 2008.
5. Price RD, Berry MG, Navsaria HA. Hyaluronic acid: the scientific and clinical evidence. J Plast Reconstr Aesthet Surg 60:1110, 2007.
6. Garg HG, Hales CA. Chemistry and Biology of Hyaluronan. Oxford: Elsevier Science, 2004.
7. Haney AF, Doty E. A barrier composed of chemically cross-linked hyaluronic acid (Incert) reduces postoperative adhesion formation. Fertil Steril 70:145, 1998.
8. Morali G, Polatti F, Metelitsa EN, et al. Open, non-controlled clinical studies to assess the efficacy and safety of a medical device in form of gel topically and intravaginally used in postmenopausal women with genital atrophy. Arzneimittelforschung 56:230, 2006.
9. Goodman MP. Female cosmetic genital surgery. Obstet Gynecol 113:154e, 2009.
10. Goodman MP, Placik OJ, Benson RH III, et al. A large multicenter outcome study of female genital plastic surgery. J Sex Med 7(4 Pt 1):1565, 2010.
11. Vogt PM, Herold C, Rennekampff HO, eds. Autologous fat transplantation for labia majora reconstruction. Aesthetic Plast Surg 35:913, 2011.

CHAPTER 10

Complications of Female Cosmetic Genital Surgery

Christine A. Hamori

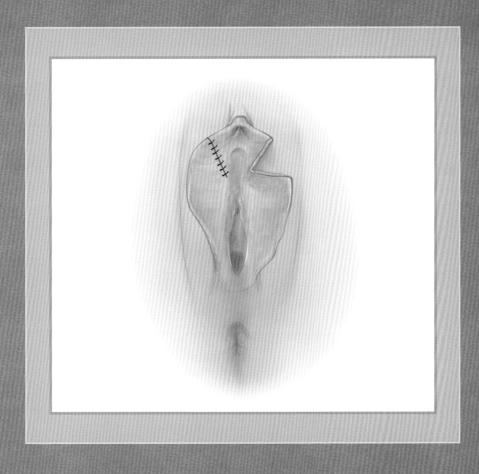

Key Points

- *Complications of cosmetic vulvar surgery are low, between 2% and 4%.[1,2]*

- *Labia minora reduction is a safe and effective surgery. Complications occur in smokers and in those with high BMIs. Edge dehiscence is the most common complication of both linear resection and wedge resection.*

- *Large hematomas are rare but require surgical drainage in the operating room. Smaller hematomas resolve with time but cause bruising and pain.*

- *Various complications such as scar widening, fenestrations, "coin slot," webbing, and pigment mismatch may occur with the wedge technique.*

- *Edge trim complications include contour irregularity, amputation, and "penis deformity."*

- *Fat grafting and fillers to the mons pubis and labia majora restore volume but may require more than one treatment. Fat necrosis is uncommon but may occur.*

- *Labia majora reduction complications include scar visibility and vaginal gaping. Conservative resection and tension-free closure will prevent these problems.*

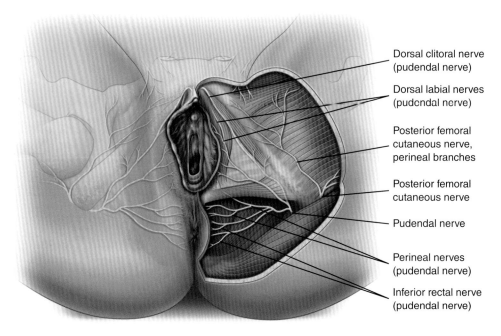

Dorsal clitoral nerve
(pudendal nerve)

Dorsal labial nerves
(pudendal nerve)

Posterior femoral
cutaneous nerve,
perineal branches

Posterior femoral
cutaneous nerve

Pudendal nerve

Perineal nerves
(pudendal nerve)

Inferior rectal nerve
(pudendal nerve)

Fig. 10-1 Superficial and deep nerves of the female perineum.

In general, complications of cosmetic vulvar surgery are low, between 2% and 4%.[1,2] The neurologic structures are quite deep and well collateralized (Fig. 10-1). Complications vary depending on the procedure. Because labiaplasty is the most common female aesthetic procedure performed, information about complication rates primarily pertain to labia minora reductions. In a review of 407 labia minora reductions, Alter[2] reported an overall reoperation rate of 2.9%.

Labia Minora Reduction Complications

Wedge Resection Complications

Labia minora reduction is a safe and effective technique to reduce the size and protrusion of the labia minora. Complications can occur, and surgeons must be adept in handling them. Complications of wedge labiaplasties that require revision occur in 4% of cases.[2,3] These include hematoma, edge dehiscence, fenestrations, pigment mismatch, and scar widening (Figs. 10-2 through 10-6). Patients who develop wound-healing problems usually present with high BMIs or have a history of smoking. The linear edge resection technique may be a better choice in these patients. Wound complications from edge trim procedures are less common in general.

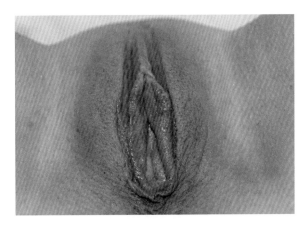

Fig. 10-2   This 33-year-old smoker is shown 8 weeks after wedge labiaplasty with right webbing (partial dehiscence).

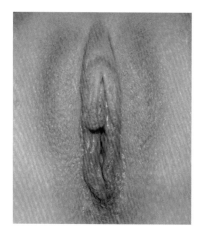

Fig. 10-3   This 22-year-old smoker, shown 4 months after a wedge labiaplasty, has a large, right notch deformity.

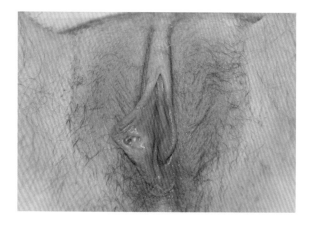

Fig. 10-4   This 18-year-old smoker, shown 8 weeks after a wedge labiaplasty, has a fenestration.

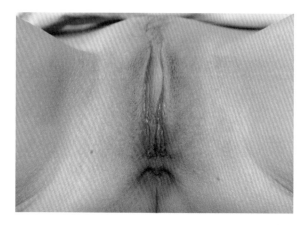

Fig. 10-5   This 42-year-old patient, shown 2 years after a wedge labiaplasty, has scar widening and pigmentation stepoff.

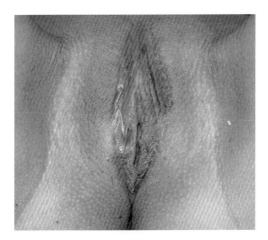

Fig. 10-6 This 25-year-old smoker, shown 4 months after a wedge labiaplasty and labia majora reduction, has pigment mismatch, scar widening, edge webbing, and narrowing of the introitus.

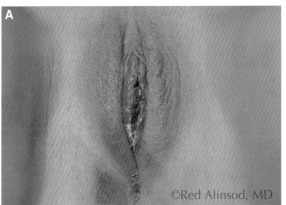 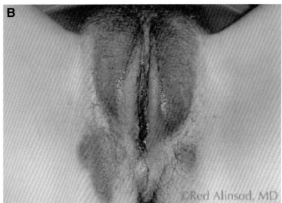

Fig. 10-7 Day 1 postoperative images of two patients. **A,** Mild bruising. **B,** Moderate bruising.

Bruising and Hematomas

Postoperative bruising is common during the first week after labiaplasty. Those prone to bruising may take *Arnica montana* around the time of the procedure to help reduce the duration of the discoloration. True hematomas are rare among postoperative perineal surgical complications (Fig. 10-7). Smaller hematomas present with pain, localized swelling, and tenderness. Patients frequently are frightened and anxious to know if surgical intervention is necessary. Using a cell phone camera, patients can take a snap shot of the area and send it to the surgeon, who can use it to help determine the course of action. Small hematomas usually get absorbed, but sometimes the dark "crank case oil" (colored fluid) may ooze from the incision several days or even weeks later. Patients should be informed of this possibility if a hematoma is noted in the physical examination. Labia minora hematomas are usually unilateral, which may cause concern for patients regarding asymmetry. Reassurance is necessary to alleviate fears of a persistent deformity. Icing, pressure, and close observation for the enlargement of the lesion are the main treatments.

Large hematomas usually form within the first 24 hours of surgery (Fig. 10-8). In my experience, surgical hematomas occur more frequently after labia majora reduction. The fascial planes of the perineum and potential spaces of the vulva allow large amounts of blood to accumulate before bleeding is tamponaded (Fig. 10-9). These cases need to be treated promptly with the patient under general anesthesia. After the clots have been irrigated and hemostasis obtained, suction drain catheters should be placed to prevent seroma formation. Once the drains are removed and the swelling decreased, a good cosmetic outcome is possible.

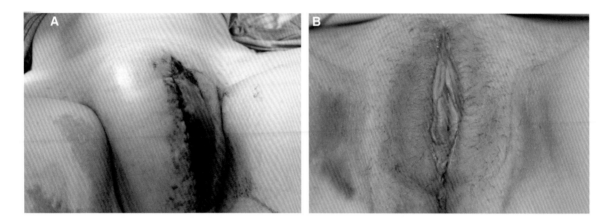

Fig. 10-8   A, This 24-year-old female has a large hematoma 8 hours after a labia majora reduction. **B,** Two weeks after drainage of the large hematoma.

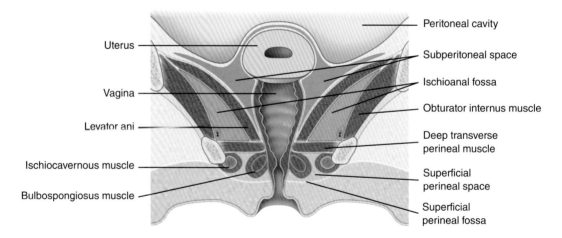

Fig. 10-9   The perineal muscles and potential spaces.

Edge Dehiscence

The most common complication for the wedge technique is an edge dehiscence or notch deformity.[2] These are seen most frequently in smokers and obese patients. Careful preoperative counseling on smoking (complete cessation of smoking 8 weeks before surgery) and weight management should be part of the preoperative management of labiaplasty patients.

Edge dehiscence or notching usually occurs at the most distal edge of the wedge closure (see Fig. 10-3). The mucosal edges tend to invert, thus preventing submucosal approximation and proper healing. Interrupted buried sutures of 4-0 Monocryl placed in the dermis of the wedge defect significantly decrease the incidence of edge dehiscence and webbing. Tension on the closure is another cause of dehiscence; thus conservative wedge resection is important. The anterior and posterior labial remnants must approximate with little or no tension. A vertical mattress suture of 5-0 Monocryl along the leading edge helps to reduce the incidence of notching and dehiscence.

For patients in whom dehiscence is a concern, such as smokers and obese patients, performing an edge trim as opposed to a wedge technique may be prudent. An edge trim does not create as deep a wound as the wedge technique. Thus, if wound-healing problems develop, the resulting wound to close by secondary intention is smaller. Wedge dehiscence is usually treated by edge reduction (trimming the protrusive segments to match the baseline of the dehisced segment), as opposed to repeating a wedge resection, which has a very high recurrence rate.

Scar Widening

Scars in wedge labiaplasty generally heal well. However, if undue tension is placed on the closure, scar widening or thickening may occur (Fig. 10-10). Reexcision of these attenuated scars is difficult, because further tissue resection results in more tension along the new suture line. Thickened scars, which very rarely occur in the labia minora, may be treated with low-dose steroid injections.

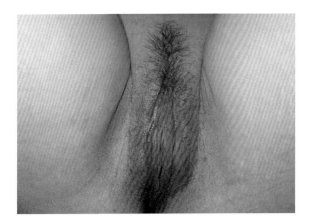

Fig. 10-10 This 24-year-old patient has scar hypertrophy 8 weeks after a labia majora reduction.

Fenestrations

Windows, rents, and webs are located more proximally along the line of wedge closure. These may occur when excess submucosal tissue is removed with the wedge (Fig. 10-11). These fenestrations also occur more often with deepithelialization labiaplasty techniques. Other causes of fenestrations include tight through-and-through sutures that can occur during wound closure that occludes vessels. Sutures should be placed with minimal tension on knot tying. To prevent complications, minimal submucosa should be removed and good dermal approximation of the remaining tissues performed. The only exception to this is in very thick labia minora, where reduction of the bulk (excess submucosa) is necessary to achieve a good aesthetic result (Figs. 10-12 and 10-13).

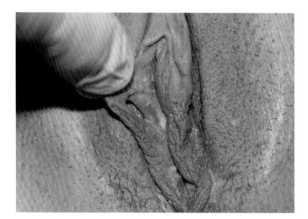

Fig. 10-11   This 30-year-old has a fenestration 8 weeks after a wedge labiaplasty.

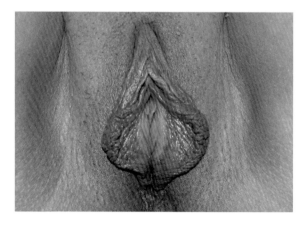

Fig. 10-12   This 49-year-old patient has thickened edge and excess submucosa.

Small edge defects or notches where adequate tissue remains may be treated with primary closure. Larger defects extending more proximally along the labial closure may be improved by trimming the remaining tissue on either side of the notch down to the level of the notch (Fig. 10-14). This modified edge trim may significantly reduce the protrusion of the labia minora and may not be warranted in cases of large proximal notches. If the dehiscence is full thickness extending to the base of the wedge closure, local flaps from the remaining labial tissue or clitoral hood may be necessary.[4]

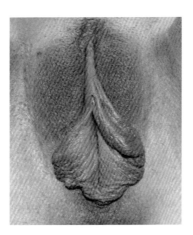

Fig. 10-13 This 22-year-old patient has thick submucosa, asymmetry, and a connected posterior fourchette.

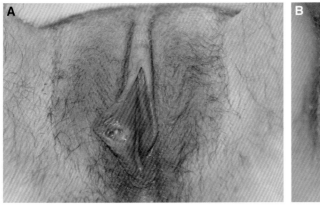 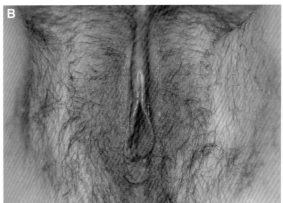

Fig. 10-14 A, This 29-year-old patient had a wedge labiaplasty and developed a fenestration, which was treated with an edge resection. **B,** She is shown 8 weeks after the edge resection.

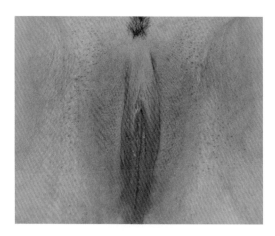

Fig. 10-15   This 30-year-old female has a coin slot appearance after undergoing a wedge labiaplasty with posterior distraction of the clitoral hood.

Coin Slot

Aggressive wedge resection of the labia may cause a tight slitlike or coin slot appearance (Fig. 10-15). The coin slot appearance is popular in coastal states such as California and Florida. Women in the adult entertainment industry specifically request the "Barbie look" (see Chapter 5). Others think that the coin slot appears unnatural. Nevertheless, removal of a too-large wedge segment may retract the clitoral hood posteriorly covering the glans clitoris. This can decrease clitoral sensitivity. Correction may involve an inverted-V incision along the dorsal hood, thereby shortening the length and restoring appropriate clitoral coverage.

Webbing

Posterior webbing may result from wedge resection in patients with confluence of the labia minora posteriorly along the posterior fourchette (see Fig. 10-13). Patients may feel rubbing and discomfort with intercourse because of posterior impingement of the introitus (Fig. 10-16). Treatment consists of a sagittal release of the web with blending of the web remnants to the posterior labia minora. Noting this anatomic variant preoperatively and performing this procedure at the time of the wedge resection can prevent this problem. Patients should be counseled preoperatively about the location of this scar. This area takes longer to heal and results in more discomfort, compared with the wedge incision.

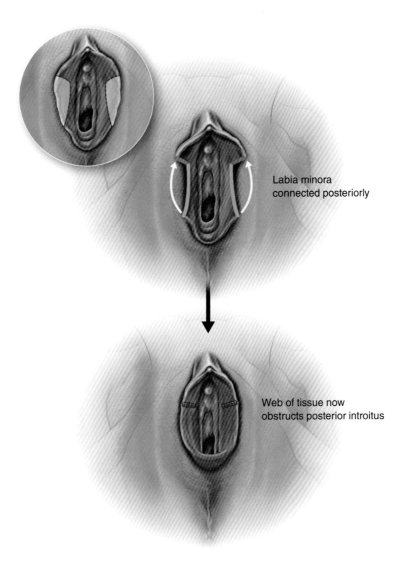

Labia minora
connected posteriorly

Web of tissue now
obstructs posterior introitus

Fig. 10-16 Posterior webbing after a wedge resection. Patients with a connected posterior fourchette or posterior lip are prone to posterior rubbing with intercourse after a wedge resection. To prevent elevation of the posterior lip with a wedge closure, the web should be incised sagittally after the wedges have been closed, creating two separate labia minora posteriorly.

Pigment Mismatch

Pigmentation patterns vary greatly in the perineal area. Labia minora tend to be most deeply pigmented along the distal arc. The wedge should be placed such that the remaining labial tissues (anterior and posterior segments) have similar pigmentation. Failure to match color along the closure site may result in an abrupt pigment change or stripe (Fig. 10-17). If pigmentation of the labia minora is bothersome to the patient, performing an edge resection should be strongly considered. A combination of a wedge and an edge trim can address segmental areas of pigmentation. Most pigment mismatches are self-resolving, but it may take 6 to 12 months for an abrupt transition to appear smooth.

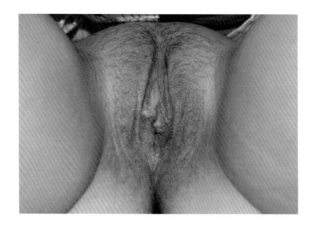

Fig. 10-17   This 23-year-old patient is shown 2 weeks after a wedge resection, with a pigment stripe along the incision site.

Treatment of a pigment mismatch or stripe is difficult. Bleaching with hydroquinone rarely achieves significant long-term improvement of the band. Further resection of the distal labia minora edge and the area of pigment mismatch may be necessary.

Edge Trim Complications

Amputation

Edge resection procedures are technically easier to perform, but complications may occur. The most common problems are related to the aggressive trimming of the free edge of the labia minora. Overresection may result in complete amputation of the labia minora. Specifically, the top third of the labia minora retracts more dramatically than the bottom two thirds, and compensation should be considered when performing markings. Surgeons need to resist the temptation to place clamps on the redundant labia minora to distract them before trimming. The pink, wet mucosa of the medial portion of the labia minora is short, compared with the keratinized pigmented tissue, which begins laterally and wraps internally. In an attempt to remove adequate edge tissue, excess mucosa may be resected and result in eversion of this tissue, vaginal dryness, and discomfort with intercourse.

Penis Deformity

Patients with large clitoral hoods who undergo edge trim procedures may have excess protrusion of the clitoral hood postoperatively (Fig. 10-18). Patients may state that they see "a penis" in this area when they look in the mirror. Edge trim techniques do not reduce the anterior projection of the clitoral hood as wedge procedures do. A large hood and partially amputated clitoral frenulum become more evident after labial edge trim

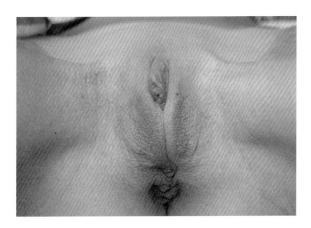

Fig. 10-18 This 41-year-old patient with a penis deformity is shown 10 months after aggressive edge resection of her labia minora.

and must be addressed at the time of labiaplasty. The junction of the clitoral hood and the frenulum is an aesthetically complicated anatomic area, and much attention must be paid to sculpting this transition. Prevention requires proper intraoperative anchoring of the confluence of the clitoral hood and labia minora when an edge trim is performed.[5]

Correction of the prominent clitoral hood as a result of aggressive edge trim consists of reducing the clitoral hood and displacing the hood posteriorly to a more anatomic position. This may be done by wedge resection if minora remnants are adequate or by reanchoring the confluence of the clitoral hood and minora to a more posterior position.

Fat Grafting and Augmentation Complications

Fat grafting to the mons pubis and labia majora can revolumize the area, which gives it a more youthful appearance. As with other areas of the body, fat integration and longevity can vary. Patients need to be informed that a second session of fat grafting may be necessary 6 to 8 months after treatment. Fat necrosis that results in lumps and cysts is uncommon if proper technique is used (that is, the Coleman technique, which involves small cannulas and slow injection). In the case of persistent fat necrosis and inflammation, surgical excision of the grafts may be necessary.

Hyaluronic acid fillers and calcium-based fillers are effective for volumizing the labia majora. These treatments may be expensive because of the volume of product necessary to volumize the area (three to eight syringes). Complications include bruising and pain on injection. Asymmetry after filler resorption can be a problem and requires more injections for correction. Hyaluronic acid fillers are advantageous, because they may be dissolved with hyaluronidase if too much has been placed in the majora. No cases of filler embolization have been reported, but large subcutaneous vessels that are deep to the dermis may be at risk.

Labia Majora Reduction Complications

Scar Visibility

Prominent, visible sagittal scars seem to be the most common problem with labia majora reduction (Fig. 10-19). Scar placement is very important to obtain a nice cosmetic result. Hair-bearing skin begins just lateral to the intervulvar groove. The medial incision should

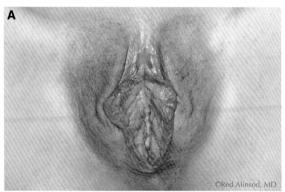
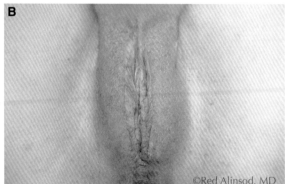

Fig. 10-19   A, This patient is shown before labia majora reduction. **B,** Postoperatively she has a prominent scar.

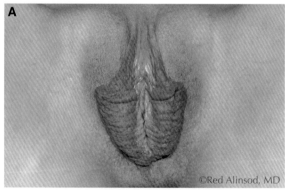

Fig. 10-20   Appropriate scar placement after labia majora reduction. **A,** Before majoraplasty. **B,** Immediately after surgery. **C,** Final result.

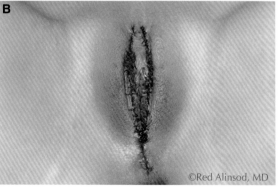
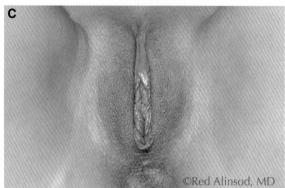

be placed just slightly internal to the hair-bearing line. Conservative resection and slight inversion or rolling of the medial flap edge with dermal sutures helps to camouflage the scar in the shadow of the majoral bulge (Fig. 10-20).

Vaginal Gaping

Aggressive resection of the majora results in splaying open of the introitus and vaginal dryness (Fig. 10-21).

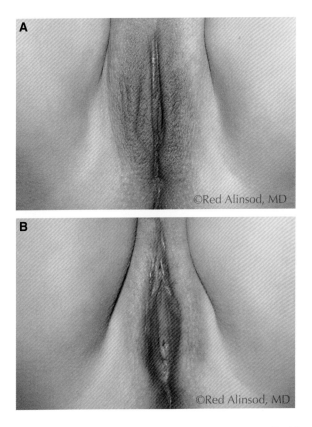

Fig. 10-21   An overresected labia majora. **A,** Before majoraplasty. **B,** After majoraplasty.

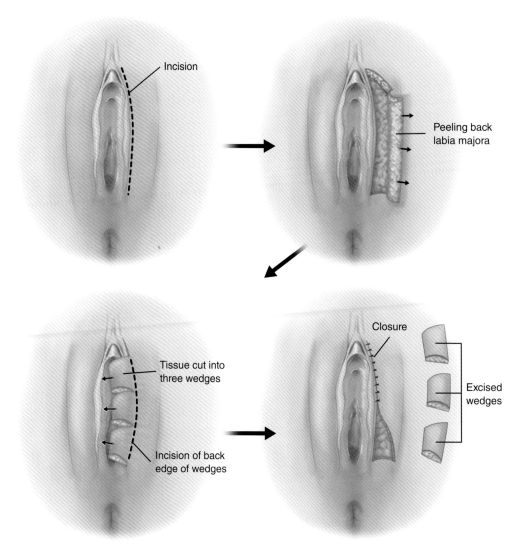

Fig. 10-22   Hawaiian skirt excision.

Overresection can be prevented by initially making the intervulvar incision medially, then dissecting laterally creating a flap. Once adequate lateral undermining is achieved, segmental skin resection is performed by bisecting the skin flap to just lateral of the medial incision. The anterior and posterior triangular flap segments are excised (Hawaiian skirt excision), and the intervulvar groove incision is closed (Fig. 10-22).

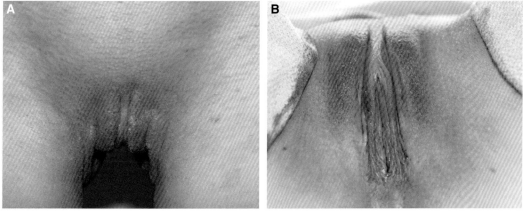

Before fat grafting

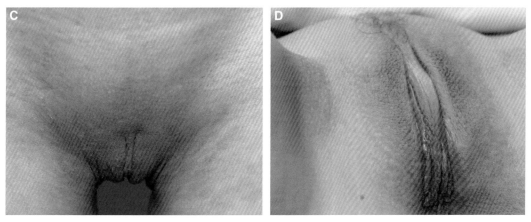

4 months after fat grafting

Fig. 10-23 **A** and **B,** This 42-year-old patient is shown before fat grafting to the labia majora and mons pubis, with 18 cc of fat injected into the mons and 12 cc injected into each labium majus. **C** and **D,** Four-month postoperative appearance.

A youthful majora is plump and rounded (Fig. 10-23), not flat and effaced. Thus conservative resection is the norm.

Secondary Procedures

Patients who have had labial surgery may have distorted anatomy from scar tissue. Careful assessment of the entire vulva is essential before proceeding with surgical intervention. The remaining labial tissues are important and usually necessitate modification to achieve the best aesthetic result. For instance, in the case of edge dehiscence in wedge resections, a combination of scar excision and trimming of remaining segments of labia minora frequently is necessary.

Scar hypertrophy in general is rare in vulvar aesthetic surgery. Labia majora scars may become widened, especially if the closure was performed under tension. Low-dose triamcinolone may be used to flatten these scars. Other options for treating visible or widened labia majora scars are either tattooing to camouflage the area or fractional resurfacing to restore pigmentation. Another option is to surgically excise the wide scars and perform a multilayer closure to minimize tension during healing.

References

1. Goodman MP, Placik OJ, Benson RH III, et al. A large multicenter outcome study of female genital plasic surgery. J Sex Med 7:1565, 2010.
2. Alter GJ. Aesthetic labia minora and clitoral hood reduction using extended central wedge resection. Plast Reconstr Surg 122:1780, 2008.
3. Goodman MP. Female genital cosmetic and plastic surgery: a review. J Sex Med 8:1813, 2011.
4. Alter GJ. Labia minora reconstruction using clitoral hood flaps, wedge excisions, and YV advancement flaps. Plast Reconstr Surg 127:2356, 2011.
5. Triana L, Robledo AM. Aesthetic surgery of female external genitalia. Aesthet Surg J 35:165, 2015.

CHAPTER 11

Perineoplasty and Vaginoplasty

Marco A. Pelosi III, Marco A. Pelosi II

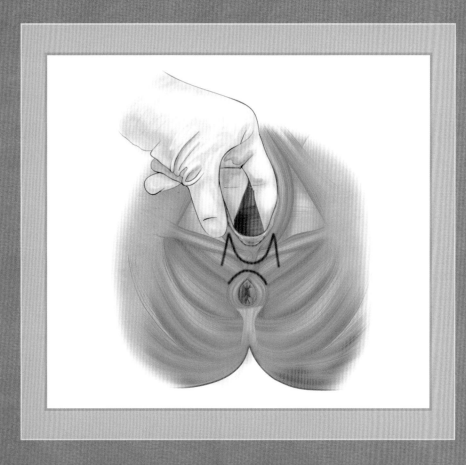

Key Points

- *Perineoplasty procedures tighten the skin and muscles of the vaginal introitus and create a convergence of the labia majora posteriorly.*

- *Colpoperineoplasty procedures tighten the skin and muscles of the lower vaginal canal and the vaginal introitus.*

- *In both procedures—perineoplasty and colpoperineoplasty—the perineal flap is carried into the subcutaneous fat layer, whereas the vaginal flap is a skin-only, superficial dissection.*

- *Transrectal digital palpation facilitates visualization and suturing of the levator muscles.*

Vaginoplasty is a general term for any procedure that reshapes the vagina. These include cosmetic and therapeutic operations of both the introitus and the canal. A few common examples are perineoplasty, vestibulectomy, cystocele repairs, rectocele repairs, colpocleisis, and colpoperineoplasty. In cosmetic gynecology, the word *vaginoplasty* has taken on a more specific connotation to refer to procedures that reduce the caliber of the vaginal introitus and the vaginal canal with simultaneous plication of the levator ani muscles.

Surgical reduction of the width of the perineum is called *perineoplasty.* Technically, it involves the excision of midline tissues spanning the perineum and lower posterior vagina and the approximation of tissues immediately lateral to the excision zone. In therapeutic gynecologic operations, perineoplasty is performed to enhance support of the pelvic floor at the time of pelvic reconstructive surgery.[1-6] In cosmetic gynecology, perineoplasty is performed to create an external muscular cuff of reduced vaginal circumference to complement a deeper zone of caliber reduction, typically executed through conservative plication of the levator ani musculature and the resection of loosened skin from the posterior vaginal wall. A secondary, purely aesthetic effect of perineoplasty is a convergence of the labia majora posteriorly (Fig. 11-1), an anatomic realignment that tightens laxity along the length of the labia majora. We take advantage of this effect when planning aesthetic procedures of the labia majora. The word *perineorrhaphy* is frequently used as a synonym for *perineoplasty.* Most practitioners use these words interchangeably, although it is linguistically incorrect to do so. The suffix *-rrhaphy* simply means "to suture," whereas *-plasty* means "to shape."

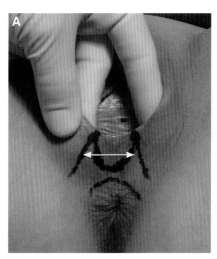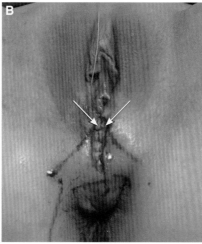

Fig. 11-1 **A,** The medial edges of the bulbocavernosus and perineal muscles are widely separated before surgery *(arrow)*. **B,** Perineoplasty causes them to converge centrally *(arrows)* to tighten the introitus and improve muscle tone beneath the labia majora.

In most instances, perineoplasty is performed as a component of colpoperineoplasty—the tightening of the vaginal canal and levator ani musculature, previously described. The most common scenario for an isolated perineoplasty is the revision of a colpoperineoplasty for a complaint of persistent laxity where only the external portion of the vaginal canal displays residual laxity. The most common misapplication of the procedure is its use in the presence of vaginal canal laxity, and the surgeon fails to recognize the diagnosis. In therapeutic gynecology, perineoplasty is sometimes used in the process of wide local excision of localized neoplasms. Many plastic surgeons use the term *external vaginoplasty* when discussing perineoplasty or even labial surgery. This is an incorrect use of the term that is common, particularly on the Internet.

Perineoplasty defines any change in the shape of the perineum, including efforts to widen the perineum and create a wider vaginal introitus. In practice, however, widening procedures are not referred to as *perineoplasty*. In these situations, we see more descriptive names such as perineal expansion, perineal release, or vestibulectomy, frequently referencing the underlying reason for the intervention.

Vaginal rejuvenation is a loose synonym for *vaginoplasty*. The popular use of the term vaginal rejuvenation in cosmetic gynecology originated in the late 1990s, when Dr. David Matlock of Beverly Hills, California, a gynecologist in private practice, coined and trademarked the term *Laser Vaginal Rejuvenation* (LVR) to market a version of colpoperineoplasty conducted with the use of a laser as a cutting instrument. A 980-diode fiber laser was used for cutting and not for shrinking tissue, as many had thought. *Vaginoplasty* is a traditional gynecologic term encompassing anterior and posterior colporrhaphies, but the lay public uses it widely to define procedures that narrow the vaginal introitus and canal.

History

The concept of tightening the vaginal dimensions altered by childbirth is not new. Vaginal rejuvenation or tightening is more than 1000 years old, and it was introduced by women.[7] The work of female physician Trotula de Ruggiero of Salerno was published in 1050 AD under the title *Treatments for Women.* The author described suturing of vaginal lacerations at childbirth, which forms the basis for all modern vaginoplasty techniques.

Also in this volume are five nonsurgical recipes for "restoring" virginity. The section opens as follows: "A constrictive for the vagina, so that women may be found to be as though they were virgins, is made in this manner."[8] Renowned Medieval historian Monica Green, who spent decades researching all extant versions of the Trotula ensemble and Salernan culture before her definitive translation, opined: "It may be that some of these constrictives were meant only to tighten the vagina to enhance the friction of vaginal intercourse, not necessarily to produce a fake bloodflow of 'defloration'; in other words, they may have been intended as aids to sexual pleasure within marriage."[8]

The Renaissance brought major advances in anatomic knowledge through cadaveric dissections. Vesalius (1514 to 1564), at the University of Padua, best represented these dissections in *De Humana Corporis Fabrica.*[9] The printing press, which was invented a century earlier, was instrumental in widely disseminating this information.

However, gynecologic surgical technique and instrumentation underwent little if any change from that of the Greco-Roman era. Nonetheless, celebrated French surgeon Ambroise Paré (1510 to 1590), in *Gynaeciorium Physicus et Chirurgicus,* and subsequently his pupil Jacques Guillemeau (1550 to 1612), in his 1609 text *De la Grossesse et Accouchement des Femmes,* were the first to describe repairs of rectovaginal lacerations at childbirth, marking the beginning of complex perineoplasty.[7]

Indications and Contraindications

Perineoplasty is indicated for tightening of the vaginal introitus only. Colpoperineoplasty is indicated for tightening of the vaginal introitus and lower vaginal canal. Rectocele, cystocele, and urinary incontinence are not treated by a perineoplasty or a colpoperineoplasty and require specific repairs, which can be performed concomitantly. Perineoplasty and colpoperineoplasty procedures should be deferred for patients who plan to have children through vaginal childbirth in the future. Patients with active infections or undiagnosed skin lesions or other pathology of the vulvar region should be treated by a gynecologist before surgery.

Patient Evaluation

Unlike medical patients who seek relief from disease, deformity, or dysfunction, cosmetic patients seeking personal or social benefits such as confidence and acceptance must be completely healthy.[10] The American Society of Anesthesiologists has developed a Physical Status Classification System for surgical patients that describes six categories: ASA I through ASA VI. Well-chosen patients are identified as ASA I or ASA II patients. These patients have no medical illness or a chronic, well-controlled medical condition. (Detailed information on the ASA system is available at *www.asahq.org*.) Hospitalization costs associated with cosmetic procedures, planned or unplanned, are not covered by conventional health care insurance.

After the initial conversation regarding the cosmetic request and the requisite psychosocial analysis, a thorough gynecologic and sexual history is obtained. This information is useful to determine whether patients have symptoms of bladder, bowel, or pelvic floor dysfunction or sexual issues that may affect treatment.

A physical examination is conducted with the patient in both a standard gynecologic dorsal lithotomy position and a standing position to fully assess for pelvic organ prolapse. A speculum examination is performed to identify any infection, which may interfere with the surgical procedure. The clitoral and bulbocavernosus sacral reflexes are assessed at the perineum. Tapping the clitoris or stroking the labia majora should produce a reflex contraction of the external anal sphincter. The patient is asked to cough to assess for bladder hypermobility. The width of the levator hiatus and the quality of the puborectalis muscle tone are assessed digitally. A common practice is to measure the hiatus in fingerbreadths with the muscles at rest and with the muscles contracted. These data are converted to centimeters. If the levator muscles are either lax or widely separated, perineoplasty alone will be insufficient to satisfy the patient's request for vaginal tightening, and colpoperineoplasty is indicated. The thickness and dimensions of the perineal body are noted. An attenuated perineal body in need of repair frequently has a thin web of skin with little to no muscular tissue. A digital rectal examination is conducted to assess for a rectocele or a perineocele, which, if present, warrants repair at the time of surgery. Rectal fullness, pressure, and constipation are very common symptoms of these conditions.

Surgeons should explain the limits of the contemplated vaginal tightening by palpating the targeted structures and by displaying the anatomy with the use of a hand mirror. Markings are useful to define the boundaries of proposed treatments and to show untargeted structures at consultation and at surgery. Dilators and fingers are used as aids to help patients visualize the degree of planned tightening. A discussion of the degree of tightness after surgery is essential.

A complete, documented medical evaluation should precede surgery in patients who have not had a recent examination. Any anatomic distortion that may increase the risk of injury should be assessed and managed by appropriate means preoperatively. Blood analyses include testing for signs of infection, anemia, and coagulopathy. Pregnancy testing is performed or repeated on the day of surgery regardless of the history.

Medications, supplements, herbs, and other substances that could impair coagulation (for example, vitamin E, gingko biloba, ibuprofen, and statins) should be discontinued 1 week in advance of surgery. Substances that interact negatively with anesthetic agents, healing, and perioperative medications should also be withheld. If they cannot be discontinued or substituted, the surgical plan will need to be modified, delayed, or withheld. Cigarette smoking is not a contraindication to perineoplasty.

Expectations and motivations need to be explored in depth in cosmetic patients. Unrealistic expectations will never be fulfilled by surgery even if procedures are performed to perfection by any medical or aesthetic standard. Cosmetic surgery "addicts," "perfectionists," and patients expecting cosmetic surgery to remedy interpersonal conflicts are examples of misguided personality types to be screened at the initial consultation.

The degree of planned tightening should be emphasized, the risks of overtightening should be explained thoroughly, and revision policies should be clearly explained.

Preoperative Planning and Preparation

Preparation for cosmetic vaginal surgery is straightforward. Acceptable results of blood analyses are confirmed. Patients should present for surgery rested and well hydrated. If sedation or general anesthesia is planned, patients are advised to not take anything by mouth for 8 hours before surgery. Informed consent is obtained, postoperative medications and wound care instructions are reviewed, and contact information is updated as necessary.

Surgical Technique

Anesthesia

Perineoplasty may be performed with local anesthesia with or without sedation, with epidural anesthesia, or with general anesthesia. Each modality has advantages, disadvantages, inherent risks, and suitability for the unique demands of each operation and patient. In our practice, perineoplasty patients are given a local anesthetic unless other procedures that warrant a different type of anesthesia are performed at the same time. Regardless of the technique, the surgical team should be knowledgeable and prepared, and the facility should be equipped to manage all potential adverse drug effects.

Tumescent local anesthesia (TLA), commonly used for liposuction, is an excellent, long-acting anesthetic for aesthetic vaginal surgery and has hemostatic properties.[10] TLA consists of lidocaine hydrochloride (800 mg/L), sodium bicarbonate (10 mEq/L), and epinephrine (1 mg/L) diluted in normal saline solution. It is injected directly into the surgical site sufficiently to cause local vasoconstriction. Typically 30 to 60 ml of TLA is sufficient and produces an anesthetic effect that lasts 8 to 12 hours. Other popular local anesthetics include bupivacaine (Marcaine and Exparel) with epinephrine and ropivacaine (Naropin) with epinephrine.

Perioperative Care

Prophylactic broad-spectrum antibiotics are routinely given immediately before surgery. Patients are placed in a dorsal lithotomy position with the legs supported in boot-type stirrups and the knees mildly flexed. Intermittent pneumatic compression stockings are routinely employed. Indwelling bladder catheterization and vaginal packing are not typically used during perineoplasty. When a colpoperineoplasty is performed, a transurethral bladder catheter and vaginal packing are maintained postoperatively for 24 hours.

Perineoplasty Technique

Markings

The procedure begins with marking of the desired diameter of the vaginal introitus. The surgeon inserts two fingers of the nondominant hand into the vagina while using the dominant hand to compress the labia majora together in the midline underneath the fingers. The uppermost contact point between the two sides is marked, and oblique lines are extended outward from the contact point for reference (Fig. 11-2).

The anterior margin of the external anal sphincter is marked. This designates the posterior limit of the surgical field. Extending the field into the sphincter proper is unwarranted and will cause increased postoperative discomfort.

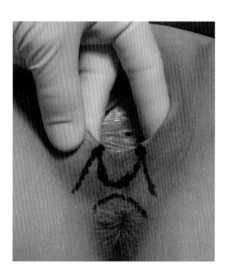

Fig. 11-2 Markings of the perineal U flap are bordered inferiorly by the external anal sphincter and bilaterally by the level of desired contact between the labia majora.

The perineal excision zone is marked as either a U- or V-shaped pattern within the bounds of the previous markings. The arms of the U or V should be wide enough to allow access to the bulbocavernosus muscles beneath the skin surface. This minimizes the need for additional dissection later and generates a more efficient dissection.

Local Anesthesia

TLA is injected whether the procedure is performed with the patient under local or general anesthesia. The main benefits are hemostasis and long-acting analgesia. It is injected with a spinal needle (18-gauge) connected to a syringe. When local anesthesia is the only agent given, the skin is first infiltrated with a small wheal of TLA, using a small needle (30-gauge) to eliminate the sensation of the larger needle.

The perineum is infiltrated with TLA in either a single left-to-right pass or in separate left-sided and right-sided passes depending on the contours and tissue dynamics. The posterior lower vaginal wall is infiltrated subcutaneously parallel to the surface in a fanning pattern while downward digital pressure is applied with the fingers of the nondominant hand.

Perineal Incision

The perineal U or V incision will extend internally to the hymenal ring. Clamps are applied to the hymenal ring at the incisional targets for maximal control (Fig. 11-3, *A*). The incision is carried deep into the subcutaneous fat to create a flap of even thickness (Fig. 11-3, *B*). The incision can be made with any instrument of the surgeon's choice. We prefer scalpel incisions, scissors undermining, and electrosurgical hemostasis at this stage.

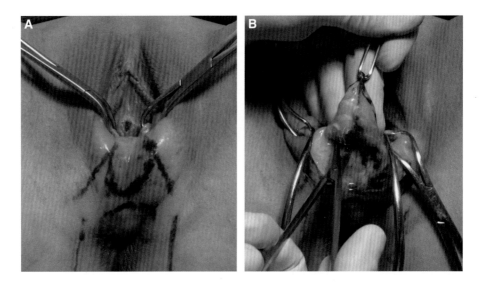

Fig. 11-3 A, Clamps mark the superior (proximal) limits of the perineal U flap at the level of the hymenal ring. **B,** The perineal U flap is raised with a thick layer of subcutaneous fat. Scar tissue is visible within the flap.

Rectovaginal Space Incision

Identification and entry into the rectovaginal space is essential for proper development of the lower vagina and for prevention of rectal wall injury. The rectovaginal space is entered most easily by retracting the perineal flap, pressing the fingers of the nondominant hand against the flap, and advancing with scissors dissection against the pressure of the fingers (Fig. 11-4). Placing the introitus on bilateral outward traction with the use of a Gelpi retractor or Allis clamps facilitates dissection. Once the dissection is at the level of the hymenal ring clamps, the rectovaginal space will have been reached. The dissection is widened until all of the superficial skin between the clamps has been undermined.

Vaginal Flap Incision

A triangular pattern is marked from the hymenal ring clamps, directed internally toward the midline (Fig. 11-5). The length of the triangle should be similar to that of the perineal flap. The vaginal flap is undermined with scissors against digital pressure from the

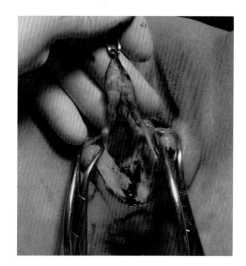

Fig. 11-4 The rectovaginal space is entered at the level of the hymenal ring by continuing the dissection subcutaneously along the posterior vaginal wall. Placing counterpressure with the nondominant hand aids the dissection.

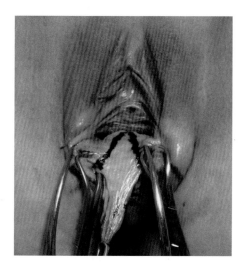

Fig. 11-5 The lower vaginal V flap is marked similar in size to the perineal U flap. It is raised as a skin-only flap. For a perineoplasty, this is the final step of dissection. For a colpoperineoplasty, the posterior vaginal wall is undermined extensively beyond the V flap, and the flap is extended superiorly.

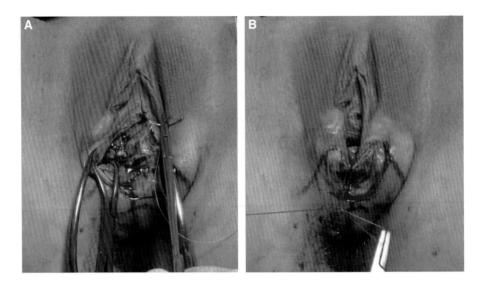

Fig. 11-6   A, After the vaginal flap is excised, the vaginal incision is closed beginning at the apex with closely spaced running sutures. **B,** The vaginal incision closure ends at the hymenal ring.

nondominant hand, as in the previous step. Having an assistant retract the apex of the triangle with an atraumatic clamp is helpful. Once the flap has been completely undermined, it is excised. No additional dissection is necessary unless a colpoperineorrhaphy is planned. If the TLA was properly injected and the dissection was properly conducted, the surgical field should be bloodless.

The surgical field is irrigated with saline solution. If the integrity of the anterior rectal wall is in question, a digital rectal examination is performed.

Vaginal Closure

Starting at the apex of the vaginal incision, a running, nonlocking delayed-absorbable suture is used to approximate the posterior vaginal wall down to the level of the hymenal ring (Fig. 11-6). Symmetry is maintained throughout while ensuring the distance between needle passes is short.

Perineal Closure

The bulbocavernosus muscles are identified. The labium majus is held between the fingers of the nondominant hand, and traction is applied to the visible incised muscle tissue with a clamp (Fig. 11-7, *A*). A proper purchase of the muscle should transmit tension to the labium majus. If no tension is felt, the clamp should be adjusted. The clamped tissue is purchased with a suture needle, the clamp is removed, and the process is repeated contralaterally to approximate the bulbocavernosus muscles with two or three interrupted delayed-absorbable sutures (Fig. 11-7, *B* and *C*). Wide (lateral) purchases of the bulbocavernosus muscles should not be performed, because they will place excess tension on the perineum. Next, the transverse perineal muscles between the bulbocavernosus muscles and the anal sphincter are identified (Fig. 11-7, *D*). These are approximated with two or three interrupted delayed-absorbable sutures (Fig. 11-7, *E*). The skin is closed in two layers—subdermal running, then interrupted skin—with fine delayed-absorbable sutures to conclude the procedure.

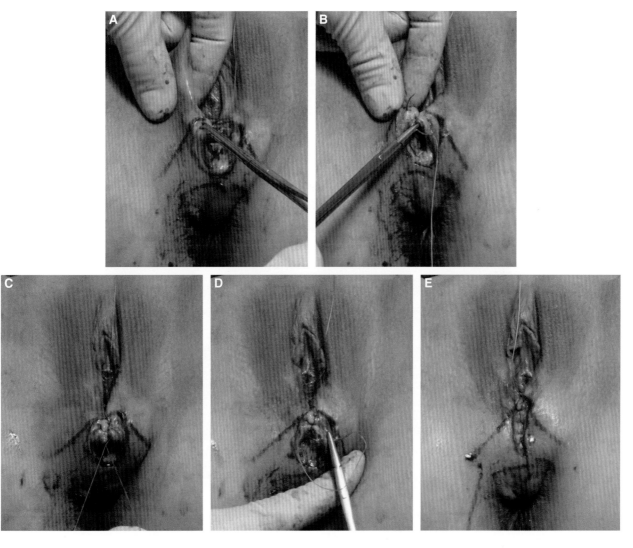

Fig. 11-7 A, The right bulbocavernosus muscle is identified with a clamp. Traction on the clamp will be palpable along the length of the right labium majus when properly applied. **B,** The clamp is removed and replaced with a "crown stitch" suture to approximate the right and left bulbocavernosus muscles in the midline. **C,** Two or three interrupted sutures are placed to reinforce the bulbocavernosus muscle plication. **D,** The transverse perineal muscles are immediately posterior to the bulbocavernosus muscles and are plicated next. **E,** Two or three interrupted sutures at the transverse perineal muscles complete the muscle plication of the perineoplasty. The skin is closed.

Colpoperineoplasty Technique

A colpoperineoplasty is essentially a perineoplasty with the addition of an extended posterior vaginal wall dissection and plication of the levator ani musculature in the midline. The initial steps of perineal flap dissection are identical, as are the final steps of vaginal and perineal closure. The technical description will begin with the posterior vaginal flap dissection.

Extended Vaginal Flap Incision

In contrast to the vaginal V flap dissection used in a perineoplasty, the posterior vaginal wall dissection of a colpoperineoplasty is performed through a midline incision, and the V is resected from the right and left sides of the midline incision after the levator ani muscle plication has been completed. The proper avascular rectovaginal plane is dissected more efficiently when approached through a midline incision than through the edge of a resected V.

A typical approach begins with excision of the perineal U flap at its base at the level of the hymenal ring. The posterior vaginal wall is retracted at three points: bilaterally at the hymenal ring and on the midline as far proximally as possible without losing tension (Fig. 11-8, *A*). Next, narrow scissors are advanced in the midline immediately beneath the vaginal epithelium to create a tunnel for dissection of the rectovaginal space (Fig. 11-8, *B*). The dissection is extended bilaterally as far as exposure and traction will allow, and the vaginal epithelium is divided in the midline and pulled toward the surgeon, facilitating

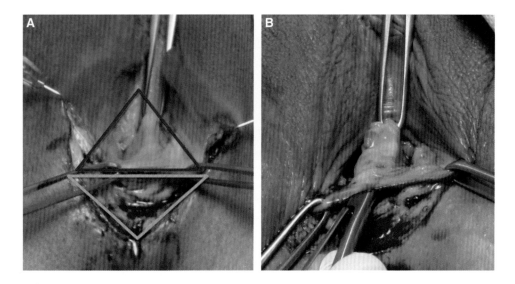

Fig. 11-8   A, The perineal flap has been resected *(blue),* and the posterior vaginal wall is retracted at three points *(red)* in preparation for dissection. **B,** Narrow scissors are advanced in the midline to create a tunnel immediately beneath the vaginal epithelium in the rectovaginal space.

further dissection superiorly and bilaterally (Fig. 11-8, *C* through *E*). When dissection through the midline has been completed bilaterally, the apical clamp is reapplied more superiorly along the midline vaginal wall, and outward traction is applied to the edges of the incised vaginal epithelium (Fig. 11-8, *F*). The process of midline subepithelial tunneling, bilateral rectovaginal dissection, and midline incision is repeated.

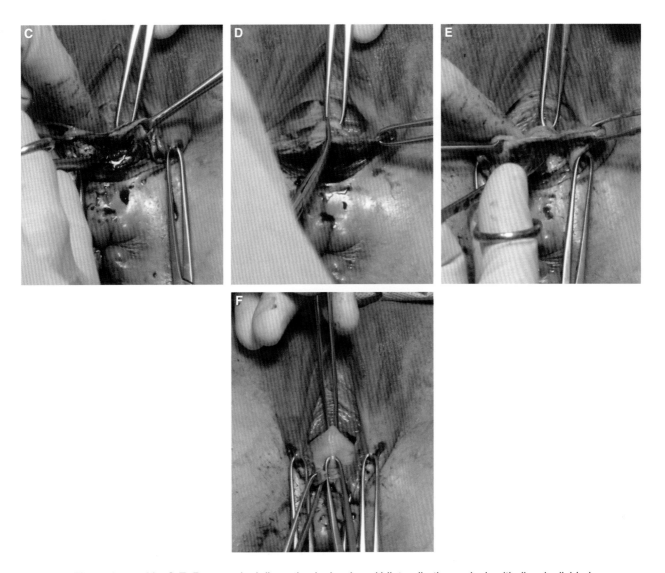

Fig. 11-8, cont'd   C-E, Rectovaginal dissection is developed bilaterally, the vaginal epithelium is divided in the midline, and traction is applied to the vaginal wall to advance the dissection further. **F,** When dissection through the midline has been completed bilaterally, the apical clamp is reapplied more superiorly along the midline vaginal wall, and outward traction is applied to the edges of the incised vaginal epithelium.

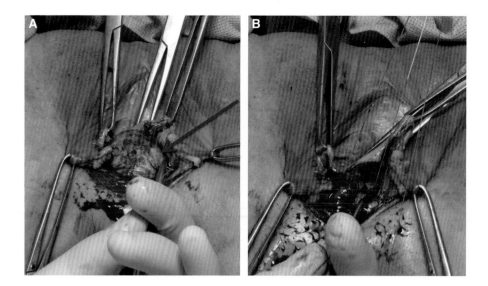

Fig. 11-9   A, Levator muscle plication suturing begins on the medial edge of the left levator muscle *(arrow)* aided by transrectal digital elevation of the muscle tissue. **B,** The right and left levator ani muscles have been retracted with a single suture. Additional suturing is performed inferior to the original suture. Sutures will be placed superior to the original suture to generate the desired degree of plication.

Levator Ani Muscle Plication

At this stage, the levator muscles will be identified. The index finger of the nondominant hand is inserted transrectally and advanced laterally and upward, tenting the levator muscle into view. An assistant pulls upward on the vaginal flap on the same side to increase exposure. Any remaining connection between the muscle and the overlying vaginal flap is dissected free to ensure complete mobility at the level of the muscle. A delayed-absorbable suture is placed through the exposed muscle approximately 1 cm medial to its edge and deep enough to ensure that it will not tear out (Fig. 11-9, *A*). The procedure is repeated contralaterally with the same suture, and tension is assessed by placing traction on the suture. With traction maintained, additional sutures are placed inferiorly and superiorly as needed to generate the desired degree of apposition and tension (Fig. 11-9, *B*). A second layer of suturing is performed over the first layer for reinforcement. A V flap of vaginal epithelium is excised from the posterior vaginal wall, and vaginal and perineal closure is completed identical to that of a perineoplasty. Because of the extended dissection required for muscle plication, tight vaginal packing is placed, along with a transurethral Foley catheter attached to a leg bag. The packing is maintained overnight.

Technical Considerations

Maintaining the levator ani sutures no more than 1 cm from their medial edges prevents the creation of palpable suture bridges along the posterior vaginal wall. These are a source of discomfort during sex. This maneuver also provides excellent control over the amount of tension desired. If more tension is desired, the second row of overlying sutures can be placed as an imbrication layer to gain an additional 1 to 2 cm of apposition without creating suture bridges.

The choice of suture material varies between surgeons. However, palpable knots of firm monofilament sutures must not be used, because during sex they will feel like needles to the patient's partner. Running sutures of 2-0 delayed-absorbable monofilament are an excellent choice and minimize the need for knots in locations where they are at risk for being felt.

Postoperative Care

The area is washed with surgical soap, and a vaginal pad is applied as a dressing, and the Foley catheter and vaginal pack are removed on the morning after surgery. The patient is instructed to avoid direct pressure to the suture line during the first week and to avoid any vaginal insertion until healing is complete approximately 6 weeks after surgery. The patient is also instructed to irrigate the area with dilute chlorhexidine solution after voiding and bowel movements. Soaking in the tub is discouraged. Nonsteroidal antiinflammatory drugs are sufficient for analgesia. No dietary restrictions are required. We have found that keeping the stools soft is critical to a good recovery. Daily milk of magnesia works well. We also recommend Colace and fiber products (for example, FiberCon or Metamucil), prunes, and prune juice.

The patient is examined 1 day after a colpoperineoplasty, 1 to 3 days after a perineoplasty, and 6 weeks after both procedures to assess healing and to determine whether she is ready to resume intercourse.

Results and Outcomes

Perineoplasty Example

A healthy 29-year-old athlete with no previous surgery requested vaginal tightening for treatment of a "looser feeling during sex for several years" (Fig. 11-10). She was 5 feet 5 inches tall, weighed 130 pounds, and was para 0. On examination, she had perineal laxity with intact neuromuscular reflexes, no vaginal laxity, and thick levator muscles with excellent tone. She underwent perineoplasty under local anesthesia. The total operating time was 45 minutes, blood loss was minimal, and a vaginal pad was placed over the surgical site. She was discharged home with a prescription for ibuprofen and noted excellent pain relief at an examination 24 hours later. She was fully healed by her 6-week examination, resumed sex at 8 weeks, and reported complete satisfaction with her results at her 12-week examination.

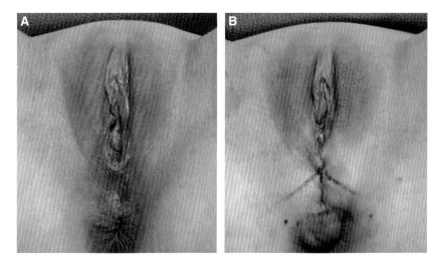

Fig. 11-10   A, Preoperative appearance. **B,** Immediately after perineoplasty, the patient has increased length of the perineal body and convergence of the labia majora posteriorly, with improved muscular tone along the labia majora.

Colpoperineoplasty Example

A healthy 35-year-old fitness model with a previous episiotomy repair requested vaginal tightening for treatment of childbirth-related vaginal laxity and labia majora augmentation for correction of age-related volume loss (Fig. 11-11). She was 5 feet 2 inches tall, weighed 110 pounds, and was para 1. On examination, she had perineal laxity and scarring with intact neuromuscular reflexes, vaginal laxity, and average-thickness levator muscles with excellent tone and a 5 cm levator hiatus. She underwent a colpoperineoplasty, liposuction of her inner thighs, and an autologous fat transfer to the labia majora. This was performed with the patient under local ancsthesia. The total operating time was 140 minutes, and blood loss was minimal. A Foley catheter, a vaginal pack, and a vaginal pad were placed at the end of her surgery. She was discharged home with a prescription for Percocet and an oral antibiotic and reported excellent pain relief on examination 24 hours postoperatively. She was fully healed at her 8-week examination, resumed sex at 9 weeks, and, in an email, reported complete satisfaction with her results shortly thereafter.

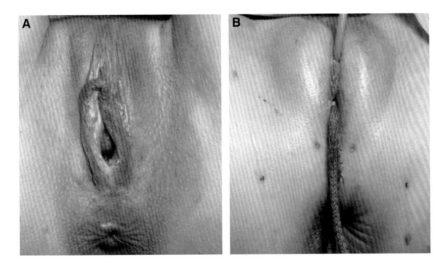

Fig. 11-11   A, Preoperative appearance. **B,** Postoperative appearance. Increased length of the perineal body and the volume and tightening effect of combining fat injections with surgical muscle tightening are obvious.

Problems and Complications

Intraoperative Complications

Intraoperative complications with a perineoplasty are exceedingly rare and are usually limited to rectal injury from improper dissection of the vaginal flap. Although we have not had to repair a rectal wall injury during a perineoplasty, we recommend following the same principles and strategies employed for rectovaginal injuries at the time of vaginal childbirth: (1) the tissues around the defect are mobilized with sharp dissection, while the nondominant index finger remains in the rectum to provide guidance until the edges of the defect are free of tension from surrounding tissues; (2) the surgical field is frequently and copiously irrigated with saline solution; (3) interrupted imbricating sutures (3-0 Vicryl on a tapered needle) are placed across the defect; and (4) a running imbricating layer is placed over the first layer, mobilizing the tissue as needed for a tension-free repair. Delayed-absorbable sutures are used. The surgeon continues with the perineoplasty. Oral stool softeners and antibiotics (for example, cephalexin or another second-generation cephalosporin) are prescribed for the first week after surgery.

Postoperative Complications

Bacterial infection of the surgical site is surprisingly rare with cosmetic vaginal surgery despite the proximity of the anus and the frequency of bowel movements adjacent to the surgical site. The most common organisms are bowel flora. Wound cultures may help to direct appropriate antibiotic therapy but should not delay management, which involves standard principles of wound care.

Yeast infections precipitated by antibiotics given at the time of surgery are more typical. These can be diagnosed visually quite easily because of the associated white, lumpy discharge. Patients often report itching. These infections are treated effectively with oral antifungal agents.

Cystitis and urethritis sometimes develop after vaginal surgery, are not difficult to diagnose, and are readily treated with oral antibiotics. The symptoms include suprapubic cramps, burning with urination, and urinary frequency. The diagnosis is made by urinalysis, and treatment includes oral sulfamethoxazole/trimethoprim (Bactrim). Urinary retention, although quite rare in perineoplasty patients, sometimes occurs after colpoperineoplasty procedures and can cause severe discomfort if not managed promptly with an indwelling urinary catheter for 24 hours.

Wound dehiscence, usually partial, can occur with trauma to the perineum during the early healing phase. Treatment is prompt surgical repair using the same steps performed in the initial closure. This heals well. Tension high enough to prevent reapproximation is highly unusual. If it occurs, frequent cleansing of the area with dilute chlorhexidine gluconate solution (2% to 4%) and the application of a thin dressing of Vaseline will expedite the formation of healthy granulation tissue until the wound is repaired. The risk for fistula is not increased by dehiscence of the surgical scar, because the surgery does not involve the rectal wall.

Pain from an overaggressive perineoplasty can be managed with either the extended use of vaginal dilators or a perineal release. The release consists of making a vertical incision through the center of the perineoplasty scar sufficient to release tension and suturing the left and right sides of the incision independently. It can be performed effectively with the patient under local anesthesia.

Pain from an overaggressive levator ani plication can be managed in one of two ways. The first, a nonsurgical option, is the injection of botulinum toxin type A directly into the levator muscles bilaterally at the site of plication. This is facilitated by transrectal digital counterpressure. The dosage is dependent on the amount of muscle tissue involved and the degree of tension present. A reasonable initial dose is 50 to 100 units divided bilaterally across the area of overplication. The second treatment option is a surgical release. This is performed through a transverse incision across the vaginal introitus to enter the rectovaginal space. The vaginal epithelium is sharply undermined to the level of the constricted tissue, and a vertical incision is made through the constricted tissue while the depth of the incision is palpated transrectally.

Conclusion

A perineoplasty is a straightforward procedure that effectively reduces the caliber of the vaginal introitus and provides a thick bridge of muscular tissue that enhances vaginal tightening in combination with a colpoperineoplasty. It results in an aesthetic convergence of the labia majora posteriorly as a secondary benefit.

References

1. Mouchel T, Mouchel F. Basic anatomic features in perineology. Pelviperineology 27:156, 2008.
2. Lewicky-Gaupp C, Fenner DE, DeLancey JO. Posterior vaginal wall repair: does anatomy matter? Contemp Ob/Gyn 54:44, 2009.
3. Petros PE. The integral theory system: a simplified clinical approach with illustrative case histories. Pelviperineology 29:37, 2010.
4. Reid R. Recto-enterocoele repair: past problems and new horizons. Pelviperineology 26:9, 2007.
5. Pardo J, Solà V, Ricci P, et al. Colpoperineoplasty in women with a sensation of a wide vagina. Acta Obstet Gynecol Scand 85:1125, 2006.
6. Moore RD, Miklos JR. Vaginal reconstruction and rejuvenation surgery: is there data to support improved sexual function? Am J Cosmet Surg 29:97, 2012.
7. Pelosi MA III. The history of cosmetic vaginal surgery: part II. International Society of Cosmetogynecology, The Blog. Posted 3/9/2013. Available at *http://www.iscgmedia.com/iscg-blog/the-history-of-cosmetic-vaginal-surgery-part-ii.*
8. Green MH, ed. The Trotula: An English Translation of the Medieval Compendium of Women's Medicine. Philadelphia: University of Pennsylvania Press, 2001.
9. Vesalius A, ed. De Humana Corporis Fabrica. Basel, Switzerland: Johannes Oporinus, 1543.
10. Pelosi MA III, Pelosi MA II. Liposuction. In Laube DW, Rayburn WF, eds. Cosmetic Procedures in Gynecology. Obstetrics and Gynecology Clinics of North America, vol 37, no 4. Philadelphia: Saunders Elsevier, 2011.

CHAPTER 12

Hymenoplasty

Otto J. Placik

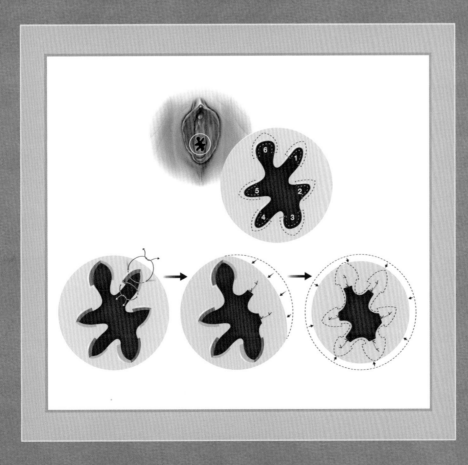

Key Points

- *Hymenoplasty is the most secretive and least studied aesthetic female genital surgery procedure.*

- *Information about the procedure tends to be based on anecdotal reports.*

- *Hymenoplasty has numerous ethical issues.*

- *Sociocultural factors play a major role.*

- *Most indications for hymenoplasty are ritualistic versus aesthetic.*

- *Establishing goals of the procedure with each patient is essential.*

- *Follow-up after hymenoplasty usually does not occur.*

- *Preoperative counseling may reduce surgical rates by 75%.[1]*

General Considerations

Hymenoplasty, which is also referred to as *hymenorrhaphy, hymen reconstruction, hymen repair, hymen restoration, hymen surgery,* and *revirgination,* is the most popular term describing surgery to reestablish the integrity of the hymen and will be used in this chapter. Of all the aesthetic female genital procedures, hymenoplasty is mired in controversy and secrecy. Although it has been classified by the World Health Organization as a type of female genital mutilation, it now is generally considered distinctly different.[2-5] Hymenoplasty is typically performed as an elective procedure; however, classifying it as an aesthetic procedure could be misleading, because others consider it more reconstructive, although nonfunctional, in nature.

Although opinions about the nature of the procedure abound, few articles discuss technical details, and data are insufficient to provide evidence to support or recommend an effective surgical approach. Patient follow-up rarely occurs, because the intended results are transient and patients prefer anonymity postoperatively.[6,7] Therefore many of the comments reported here were acquired on a personal basis during patient interactions and otherwise cannot be substantiated using traditional medical references.

It has been said that, "A woman's future can hang, literally, by a membrane."[8] Although patient safety is paramount, debate over the medical risks and practitioner skills are countered by fears of social ostracism and/or physical harm.[5,9] Central to this discussion is whether hymenoplasty should be performed at all, which essentially is a matter of ethical deliberation.[10]

Ethical and Cultural Considerations

The approach to hymenoplasty depends on the respective culture and the value it places on virginity.[3,11] Among university students in Turkey, a recent survey demonstrated the persistence of a double standard for male versus female attitudes for the traditional value of virginity that drives the demand for hymenoplasty.[12] Although many assume hymenoplasty is more popular in Islamic cultures, the procedure has been performed in other cultures around the world. For example, an estimated 2% of women in Guatemala may have received this operation, often by practitioners with questionable training and a lack of monitoring or oversight.[13]

Hymenoplasty is the most secretive and least studied aesthetic female genital surgery procedure. Information about the procedure tends to be based on anecdotal reports. The influence of religion, traditional customs, and personal beliefs may also be reflected in a particular society's legal codes.[9,14] In these countries, practitioners will offer the procedure out of a moral obligation for the safety of women requesting it, despite personal ethical reservations and the risk of punitive consequences.[15]

Although the definition of *virginity* may be contested, many people consider an intact hymen to be the sine qua non of sexual chastity.[16] For many cultures, the presence of an unbroken hymen is consistent with moral behavior and an indication of honor and integrity. I have been told stories of (1) mandatory physical examinations by "qualified" practitioners before the marriage ceremony, (2) a required breaking of an intact hymen with a cotton/silk cloth wrapped around the inspector's index finger, (3) the mother-in-law being present at the time of consummation, and (4) the proud display of the bloody sheet. In Turkey, nearly any individual with a "vested" interest can demand a hymen examination as confirmation of virginity.[17] Historically, major religions (Christianity, Judaism, Islam, Buddhism, and Hinduism) associate sexual abstinence with moral purity, and sexual activity is condoned between married individuals. Women who have had or even are suspected of premarital sexual activity (as evidenced by a compromised hymen assessed using a variety of methods that vary on a cultural basis) may be subjected to cancellation of marriage vows, public humiliation, excommunication, banishment, physical abuse, or other legal repercussions, including sentencing to capital punishment, imprisonment, or death (honor killing).[9,18,19] One report arguing for repair stated the Egyptian practice of hymenoplasty actually reduced the frequency of "cleansing" murders by 80% compared with the previous decade.[9]

The ethics committees of multiple international medical societies (United States, United Kingdom, France, Canada, New Zealand, Australia, and the World Health Organization) have generally incorporated hymenoplasty as a genital cosmetic procedure.[19-21] Goodman et al[22] have proposed the four ethical principles (patient autonomy, nonmaleficence, beneficence, and justice) that distinguish elective vulvar plastic surgery from genital cutting practices. Ethicists support physicians' decisions to perform surgery to protect women from adverse consequences.[23] Conversely, others suggest, "Gynecologists with sufficient skills asked to perform the procedure should ethically take into account the consequences of their refusal."[5] Kopelman[24] advised institution of the "Best Interests Standard" when weighing the decision to perform a hymenoplasty but thought this to be secondary to the "growing problem of forced marriages." Earp[25] suggested that physicians charge the "lowest possible fee" while combatting the greater social structure that drives the demand. Some propose that the availability of the procedure exposes a more troublesome incidence of sexual abuse, vulnerability to sexual harassment, and lack of appropriate sexual education.[14] Critics of the procedure think it can become obsolete if the public learns to accept that bleeding or hymenal examination or certificates are not confirmations of virtue.[19] Advocates have advanced elegant arguments for scientific evaluation of hymenoplasty practices and a multidisciplinary team of "surgeons, lawyers, social activists, champions of human rights, and religious leaders" to establish a solution to the controversy.[18,26]

Elective Versus Reconstructive Surgery

Rarely, I have been asked to perform an elective hymenoplasty by both partners to comply with this marriage ritual or, even more rarely, to celebrate a second honeymoon. However, it is more often requested by a female, with or without accompanying family members, to conceal any history of premarital sex from an intended future partner and to ensure the perception of virginity. This is desperately sought after to prevent the dire consequences discussed previously. The same ethical issues discussed previously apply. Within this context, many practitioners, including male and female plastic surgeons, refuse to participate in a surgical procedure that (1) is not medically necessary, (2) holds women (versus men) to a higher standard of premarital abstinence, and (3) perpetuates deception of an unknowing victim: the sexual partner.[5,7,27] One author argues that even if the bridegroom is aware, then the physician is colluding with deceit of other family members. Others question these moral arguments, given plastic surgeons' performance of breast augmentation and liposuction. These operations are similarly not disclosed to partners and are also intended to present a facsimile of a natural physical state.[22]

Some think that hymenoplasty, unlike purely cosmetic procedures such as breast augmentation, may serve a "more worthy and protective" purpose.[7] In some cultures, a "certificate of virginity" may be demanded on completion of the procedure; surgeons must be prepared to manage and address this moral conflict and their complicity in the deceit.[28] Ethicists have justified the need to provide these certificates for patients at great risk of harm to their "well-being, autonomy, or personal integrity."[29] The embarrassment of being subjected to a physical examination (for the purpose of being "officially certified" as a virgin) has caused a number of women to commit suicide.[17,19] This has prompted some advocates to suggest that partial monetary coverage should be made available when the indication is not purely aesthetic.[7]

Proponents think that the confidentiality of the doctor-patient relationship and the woman's request supersede all other concerns.[14] Others object on the basis that this maintains a prejudiced societal standard of virginity to which only women are held. Therefore condoning surgery preserves a myth that an intact hymen is a symbol of virginity. Some argue that eliminating these preconceived notions may not be a medical or legal issue and requires more of a social structural change.[17,23] Others describe it as a "ritualistic surgery" that equates with circumcision and correlate the ethics with those of cosmetic surgery.[14,18,30]

Indications and Contraindications

The function of the hymen is unknown but has been proposed as a vaginal barrier against external sources of infection until puberty.[31] Some have stated that there is, "no valid scientific indication" for hymenoplasty,[18] and that it is performed primarily for cultural indications.[8]

Nearly anyone who presents with realistic expectations and has sufficient tissue to approximate is a candidate for elective hymenoplasty. Variations in technique can be performed for patients with insufficient hymenal fragments (Fig. 12-1). The timing of anticipated coitus may play a role in selecting a surgical approach and is discussed later in the chapter. Critics of the procedure claim unscrupulous surgeons may not provide proper information to patients and encourage patients to undergo the procedure to benefit from financial incentives.[13,18]

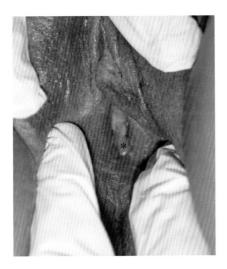

Fig. 12-1 In the examination room it is difficult to see hymenal fragments (*).

Contraindications for hymenoplasty include confusion with vaginal tightening procedures, active vulvovaginal infections, active vulvovaginal inflammatory conditions, expectations for an "idealized" hymen with a circular aperture in the center of a diaphragm, coagulopathy, and smoking.

Patient Evaluation

Clinical Evaluation of the Deformity

Although screening methods have been recommended for patients undergoing female genital plastic surgery, no established tools exist for evaluating hymenoplasty candidates.[22] The rapid healing of hymenal injuries may result in very little evidence of damage.[32] The hymen has no standard appearance; a wide variety of anatomic variations have been described.[8,33-37] Normal variations may occur with advancing age, and the hymenal morphology may change.[37-40] Studies have shown a high incidence of nonspecific findings in hymenal morphology among women without a history of sexual abuse.[41]

Moreover, the optimal hymenal diameter or size has not been determined.[42,43] Studies and discussions for establishing the "ideal" hymenal width and/or transhymenal diameter are inconclusive and summarized in an article discussing hymenal findings in females with and without a history of sexual abuse.[44] Thus, there is no standard hymenal appearance to reproduce or reconstruct.

Preoperative Planning and Preparation

Patients should be informed about the procedure with a thorough review of the risks, alternatives, and benefits consistent with the principles of informed consent.

When discussing the role and goals of the procedure, surgeons should discuss the following topics:
- Repair has no direct medical benefit.[18]
- Absence of the hymen or failure to bleed is not necessarily a sign of previous intercourse.[19]
- Less than half of the women in a retrospective survey stated they had not bled with initial sexual penetration.[45]

In a study from Amsterdam, 75% of counseled women elected not to proceed with hymenoplasty.[1] They were informed that despite expressing a desire for postcoital bleeding and assurances that they would be sufficiently "tight" on their wedding night, surgery could not guarantee either. Bleeding on first coitus does not necessarily indicate virginity, and in a survey of 41 women, only 34% of the virgins bled on first intercourse, and 63% did not.[14,46]

Determining on physical examination whether a patient has had prior sexual activity is not always possible.[47] In one study where ease of speculum examination was assessed, it was judged to be easily inserted in 56% of women who had denied sexual intercourse and had used tampons, whereas it was easily inserted in 81% of sexually active patients. The same study revealed that subjects who were not sexually active had comparable gynecologic and hymenal findings regardless of tampon (versus pad) use, sports activities, or prior pelvic examination. Nonetheless, hymenal rupture in the absence of sexual activity has been associated with prior surgery, tampon insertion, physical exercise, and masturbation.[48-50] Conversely, intact, nondisrupted hymens were reported in 52% of women who had prior sexual intercourse.[51] Bleeding may not occur, or the repair of sufficient strength may necessitate hymenotomy or surgical transection.[52]

For Muslim patients, physicians should make the distinction that although premarital or extramarital sexual relationships are strictly prohibited, proof of virginity by bleeding on the wedding night is not necessary.[19] All women (and family members) who present for restoration of the hymen with the intent to elicit postcoital bleeding as a sign of virginity, should be informed that no specific genital findings distinguish prior sexual abuse from non-abuse-related conditions.[44]

Surgical Techniques

In most reviews, the surgical technique is vaguely described, and success rates are either not reported or reported as low, with a 67% success rate in one study.[53] However, surgical approaches can be categorized as surgical flaps, surgical adhesions, lumenal reductions, suture-only techniques, or artificial membranes/reservoirs.

The timing between the procedure and coitus is a critical issue that generally receives little attention. One author discussed practitioners even performing the procedure "in the days immediately before the wedding."[54] I have learned much about it from personal communication with other practitioners. For patients who desire structural integrity and need the hymen to be intact on visual inspection, the repair should be performed 3 months before the "consummation of marital vows." However, when the timing of coitus is known, and the patient desires bleeding but visual integrity is not needed, surgery is often best scheduled 3 weeks before the date. In patients with partial wound breakdown, granulation tissue is sufficient to promote bleeding with the lightest of friction. van Moorst et al[1] suggested performing surgery no sooner than 14 days before the wedding to increase the chance of blood loss, but not much later to prevent visibility of the suture remnants.

Anesthesia, Antibiotics, and Markings

Nearly all patients have marked anxiety because of the preceding events or because they are sexually introverted; thus I advise them to have general anesthesia or monitored anesthesia care with appropriate perioperative medications. Local anesthesia with or without oral or intravenous sedation, or monitored anesthesia care, is occasionally performed for patients extremely at ease, such as those celebrating a second honeymoon, those willing to tolerate the injections, and those with time for repair. In these cases, a Telfa pad rolled into a tampon is inserted into the distal vagina. The tampon is removed immediately after the patient is positioned but before the injection and prep. The purpose of the Telfa pad is to apply pressure and direct apposition of the topical cream to the circumferential hymenal fragments rather than allow gravitational settling along the posterior wall. No controlled studies call for the use of antibiotics, but they are given in accordance with reports showing their benefits in third-degree postpartum perineal wounds.[55,56]

Patient Positioning

Patients are placed in a lithotomy position and prepped in a routine sterile fashion.

Flap Technique

Very limited discussions of the vaginal mucosal flap procedure are available and only briefly mentioned as a second option when hymenal remnants are insufficient. The description of the entire procedure is simply, ". . . a narrow strip of posterior vaginal wall is dissected for reconstruction."[14,30,57] It is rarely, if ever, performed, because it requires a repair that is sufficient to remain intact yet weak enough to rupture with penile penetration. If true squamous epithelium healing occurs, the flap may necessitate surgical release.

Surgical Adhesions

The most popular technique by far involves surgical adhesions.[57,58] However, one of the most commonly described articles cited only nine cases performed over 10 years.[46] The author based his technique on a publication mentioned in a previous publication (with 20 cases and no follow-up physical examination).[30] The surgical method was briefly mentioned in 29 words.

I have described my surgical adhesion technique in detail later in the chapter.

Lumenal Reductions

In an overview of female genital plastic surgery, Goodman[59] discussed two techniques. He reported on one method of circumferential decrease in caliber of the introitus using multiple, small, diamond-shaped excisions along the periphery of the hymenal ring and

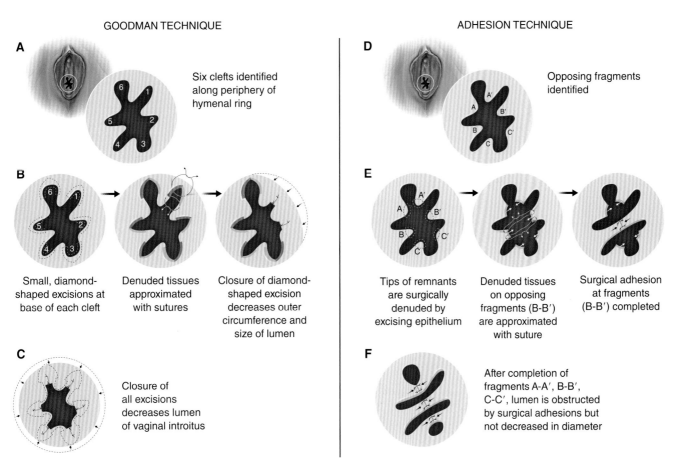

GOODMAN TECHNIQUE

A Six clefts identified along periphery of hymenal ring

B Small, diamond-shaped excisions at base of each cleft → Denuded tissues approximated with sutures → Closure of diamond-shaped excision decreases outer circumference and size of lumen

C Closure of all excisions decreases lumen of vaginal introitus

ADHESION TECHNIQUE

D Opposing fragments identified

E Tips of remnants are surgically denuded by excising epithelium → Denuded tissues on opposing fragments (B-B′) are approximated with suture → Surgical adhesion at fragments (B-B′) completed

F After completion of fragments A-A′, B-B′, C-C′, lumen is obstructed by surgical adhesions but not decreased in diameter

Fig. 12-2 A comparison of the Goodman technique and a typical technique involving denuding of opposing remnants.

the more common method of denuding opposing hymenal fragments followed by surgical adhesion.

Although the Goodman technique achieves a luminal reduction with multiple side-to-side approximations of hymenal fragments using diamond-shaped excisions between the remnants, the surgical adhesion technique results in luminal obstructions through end-to-end approximation of hymenal fragments (Fig. 12-2).

Suture-only Techniques

A variety of suture methods are available for performing a simple, expedited repair. Ou et al[60] described running a single 5-0 chromic catgut suture submucosally beneath the hymenal fragments, beginning at a puncture wound at the 6 o'clock position, extending up to and exiting the wound at the 12 o'clock position, and returning back through the same wound to the initial puncture at the 6 o'clock position. The suture is tied around a 12 mm Hegar dilator with a buried knot. Although the technique seems elegant, I have used it to reinforce traditional surgical adhesions without success. The authors reported an intact 1 cm transhymenal lumen in four of four patients examined 1 week after the procedure.

El Hennawy[8] recommended using catgut sutures to approximate hymenal remnants approximately 3 to 7 days before coitus because of the temporal nature of the procedure. He alternatively described an even easier technique of placing a transluminal suture across the hymen.

Artificial Membranes and Reservoirs

The technique of artificial membranes and reservoirs involves suturing or placing blood-like, filled gelatin capsules inside the vagina. These are intended to rupture with penile penetration, simulating tearing of an intact hymen.[9,61] Online sources provide an artificial hymen (referred to as a *Chinese hymen* or *fake hymen*) consisting of a prosthetic membrane filled with a "medical-grade red dye liquid" (comparable to human blood) that is inserted nonsurgically into the vagina.[62] The source claims that the device replicates the hymen by oozing the simulated blood on vaginal penetration. The use of alloplants has also been reported.[8]

My Technique: Modified Surgical Adhesions

Plastic surgeons are taught that optimal wound healing relies on vascularized tissues approximated with minimal wound tension. Through my experiences acquired in a plastic surgery training program, I relate my approach to that of a Furlow Z-plasty that applies these principles. The tissue handling characteristics are also comparable. The technique is described in the following steps.

1. The patient is placed in a lithotomy position and 1% lidocaine with epinephrine is injected using a 30-gauge needle. The patient is prepped and draped.
2. The labia minora are cautiously retracted with sutures or retractors to provide exposure, but with minimal tension on the introitus (Fig. 12-3, *A*).

A

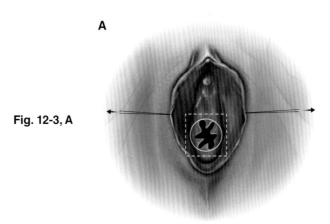

Fig. 12-3, A

Retraction of labia minora

3. The hymen is inspected for suitable opposing remnants, with a goal of completing a minimum of three adhesions (Fig. 12-3, *B*).

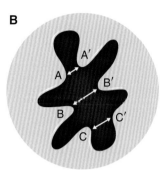

Identification of at least three
opposing remnants

Fig. 12-3, B

4. For each repair, hydrodissection of the remnant or flap is completed with 1% plain lidocaine using a 30-gauge needle to increase the size and to facilitate approximation. After the initial injection, epinephrine is not used, because these tissues are not particularly vascular, and assessment of bleeding is desired. Pressure and observation are preferred for hemostasis as opposed to electrocautery, which should be used only minimally. I prefer Gerald tissue forceps with teeth to handle tissue (Fig. 12-3, *C*).

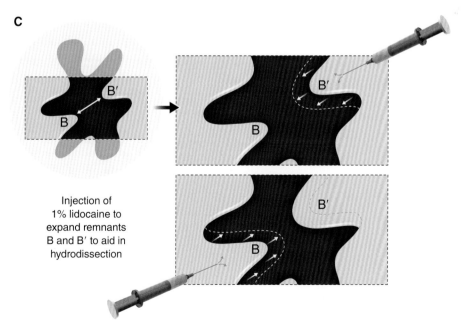

Injection of
1% lidocaine to
expand remnants
B and B′ to aid in
hydrodissection

Fig. 12-3, C

5. Once injection is complete, a No. 15C blade, a No. 11 blade, or iris scissors are used to create an anterior (distally based) flap that is unfolded, effectively lengthening the remnant. The opposing remnant is then approached, creating a posteriorly (proximally) based flap. This approach is used to reduce wound tension while increasing the surface area for healing (Fig. 12-3, *D*).

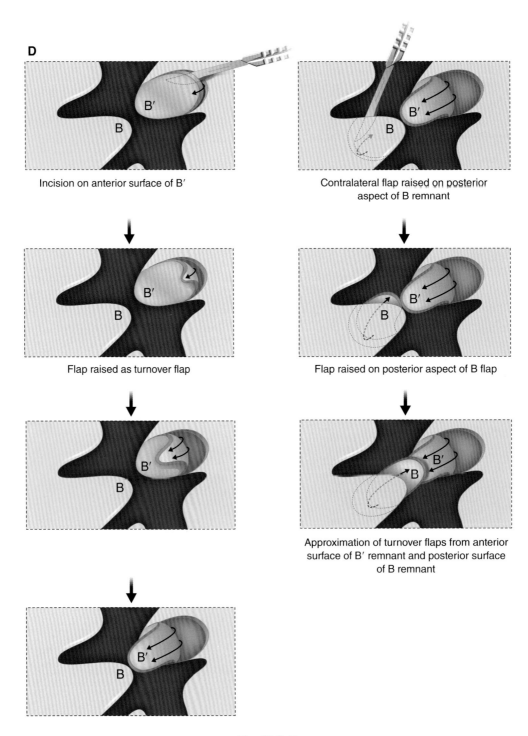

D

Incision on anterior surface of B′

Contralateral flap raised on posterior aspect of B remnant

Flap raised as turnover flap

Flap raised on posterior aspect of B flap

Approximation of turnover flaps from anterior surface of B′ remnant and posterior surface of B remnant

Fig. 12-3, D

6. If necessary the labial retraction is eased to allow coaptation (Fig. 12-3, *E*).

E

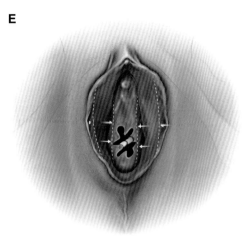

Ease retraction on labia minora so
remnants are more easily approximated

Fig. 12-3, E

7. The flaps are approximated using opposing 5-0 Monocryl sutures on RB-1 tapered needles. Occasionally, if the fragments are sufficiently thick, a buried stitch may be placed. More often, the sutures are run in a continuous simple fashion ending 180 degrees from their starting points, similar to a spatulated end-to-side vascular anastomosis (Fig. 12-3, *F*).

F

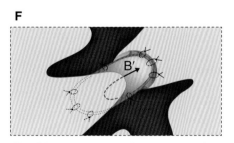

B + B′ remnant turnover flaps are sutured to
each other with 5-0 monocryl on RB-1 needle

Fig. 12-3, F

8. If bleeding occurs, pressure or observation is continued until it stops. Rarely, needle or wire-tip electrocautery is used on a low setting, but only if necessary.
9. A Telfa pad with a light application of ointment is applied.

Patient Example

Hymenal fragments are labeled. *A* will be approximated to *A′*, *B* to *B′*, and *C* to *C′*, (Fig. 12-4, *A*).

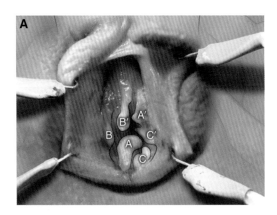

Fig. 12-4, A

Fragment *B′* is approximated to *B* (Fig. 12-4, *B*). Fragment *C* is approximated to *C′* (Fig. 12-4, *C*). Completion of the *A*-to-*A′* adhesion (Fig. 12-4, *D*).

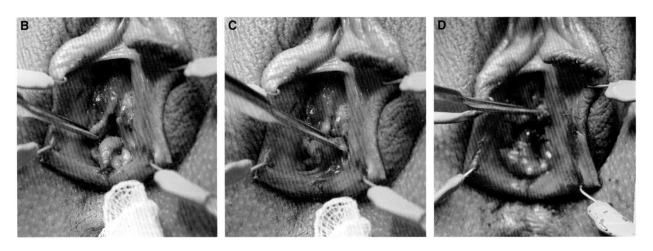

Fig. 12-4, B-D

Residual lumen is present to the right of the *A-A′* adhesion (on the patient's right) (Fig. 12-4, *E*). Residual lumen is seen to the left of the *A-A′* adhesion (on the patient's left) (Fig. 12-4, *F*).

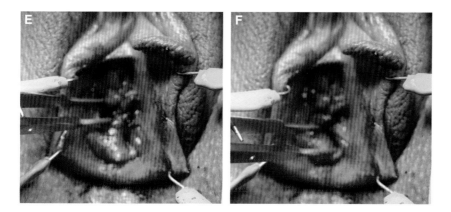

Fig. 12-4, E-F

The adhesion is simulated with a hand demonstration. The hands represent opposing hymenal fragments (Fig. 12-4, *G*). The open, upper hand represents the superior fragment being incised, which creates a flap that is turned down (the fingertips are the tip of the flap; the palm is the raw surface) (Fig. 12-4, *H*). The open, lower hand represents the inferior fragment being incised, which creates a flap that is turned and lifted upward (the fingertips are the tip of flap; the palm is the raw surface) (Fig. 12-4, *I*). The open, upper hand represents the superior flap being sutured to the inferior flap. This is represented by the open, lower hand coming to rest on the open, upper hand, with the raw surfaces approximated to each other (Fig. 12-4, *J*).

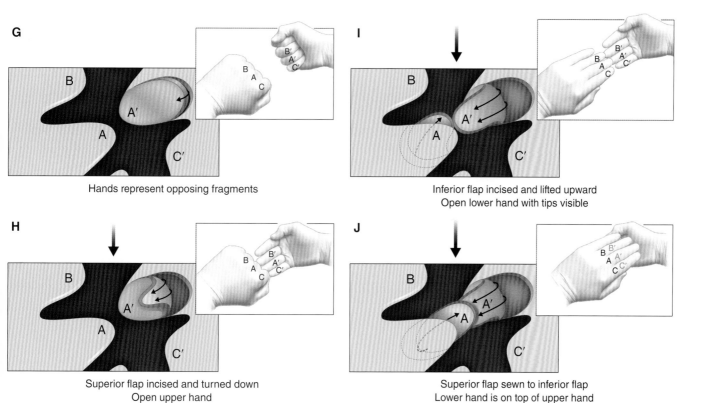

G — Hands represent opposing fragments

I — Inferior flap incised and lifted upward
Open lower hand with tips visible

H — Superior flap incised and turned down
Open upper hand

J — Superior flap sewn to inferior flap
Lower hand is on top of upper hand

Fig. 12-4, G-J

Fragment B' is incised along the anterior and distal surface to create a superiorly based turndown flap (Fig. 12-4, K). The turndown flap is shown on fragment B' as it is being incised (Fig. 12-4, L). Fragment B is incised along the posterior and proximal surface to create an inferiorly based turnup flap (Fig. 12-4, M).

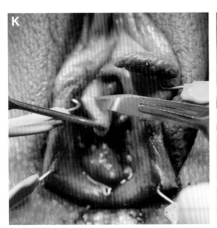
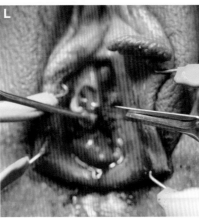
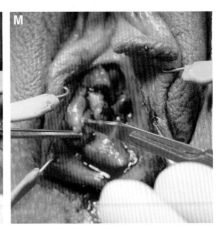

Fig. 12-4, K-M

Fragment C' is grasped before injection (Fig. 12-4, N). Fragment C' is injected to enlarge it before an incision is made and a flap created (Fig. 12-4, O). Fragment C is grasped and injected to enlarge it before an incision is made and a flap created (Fig. 12-4, P).

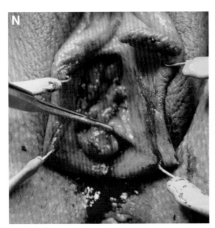
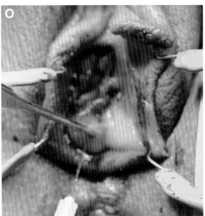
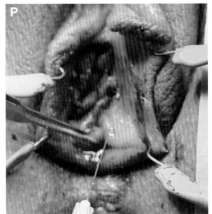

Fig. 12-4, N-P

Fragment C' is incised along the anterior and distal surface to create a superiorly based turndown flap (Fig. 12-4, Q). The turndown flap on fragment C' is shown as it is being incised (Fig. 12-4, R). Hemostasis is achieved throughout the procedure with pressure and a gauze or swab. The use of electrocautery is minimized (Fig. 12-4, S).

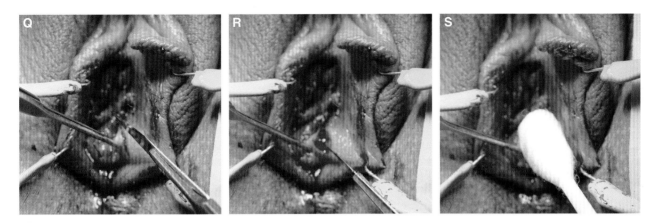

Fig. 12-4, Q-S

Suture repair of fragment *C* to fragment *C'* is shown (Fig. 12-4, *T*). 5-0 Monocryl suture with a taper RB-1 needle is used to minimize trauma to tissue typically seen with a cutting needle. Violet-colored suture facilitates visualization of the fine suture (Fig. 12-4, *U*). The three suture adhesions—*A-A', B-B'*, and *C-C'*—are labeled in Fig. 12-4, *V*. The introitus is shown after removal of the retractors (Fig. 12-4, *W*).

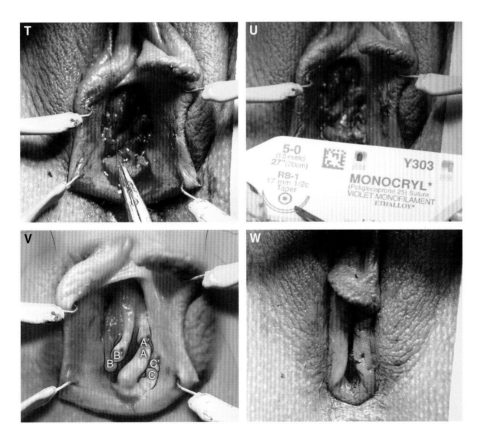

Fig. 12-4, T-W

Cerclage Technique

The operative sequence for a cerclage technique is shown in Fig. 12-5.

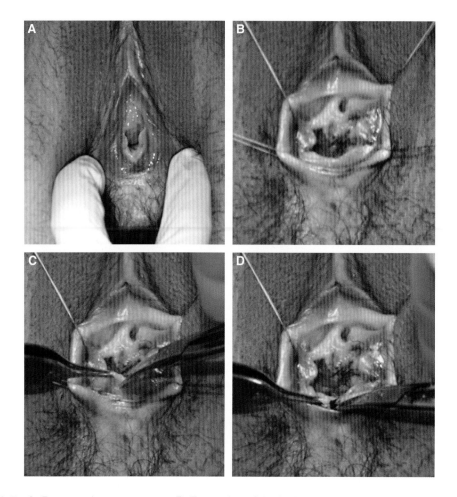

Fig. 12-5   A, Preoperative appearance. **B,** Retraction of the labia minora. **C,** An entry wound is made at the 6 o'clock position with iris scissors. **D,** The entry wound is dilated.

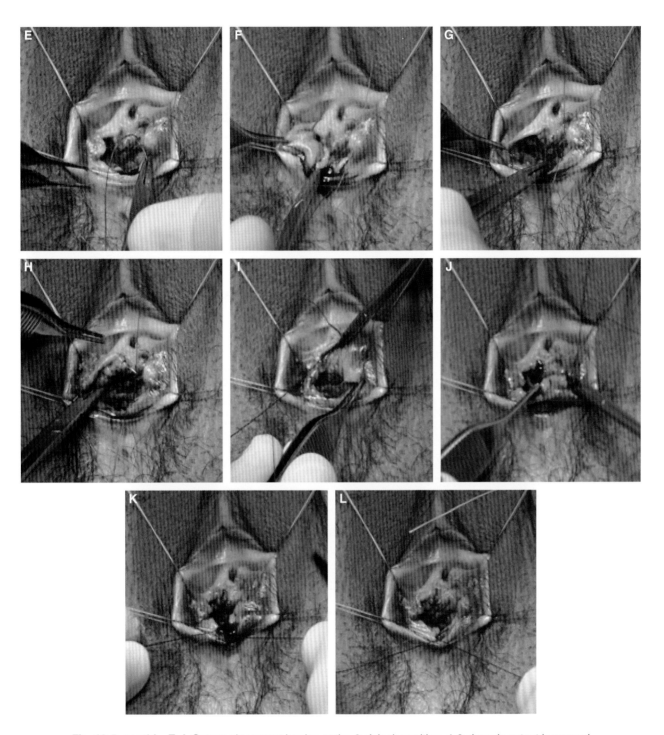

Fig. 12-5, cont'd   E-J, Suture placement begins at the 6 o'clock position. 4-0 chromic catgut is passed through the submucosa in a clockwise fashion, with exiting and reentry into each sequential puncture wound. **K,** Additional tension is applied to show the decreased size of the introitus. **L,** Suturing ends with a knot at the 6 o'clock position.

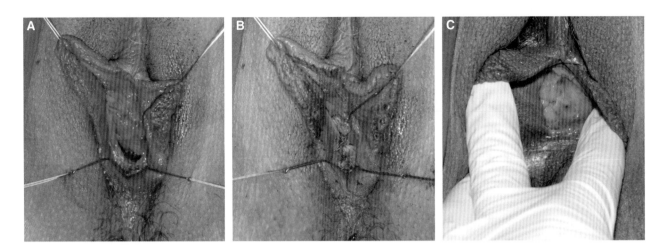

Fig. 12-6   A, Preoperative retraction shows the introitus. **B,** The patient is shown immediately postoperatively after suture approximation. **C,** Three weeks after the surgical repair, the adhesions are healed.

Traditional Technique of Denuding Flaps and Suture Approximation

The traditional method of denuding flaps with suture approximation is shown in Fig. 12-6.

Ancillary Procedures

There is a misconception that hymenoplasty will tighten the vagina, and many practitioners conflate the two procedures. With the exception of the previously described luminal reduction technique suggested by Goodman,[59] hymenoplasty does not tighten the vagina. This is discussed in Chapter 11, Perineoplasty and Vaginoplasty. The manufacturers (Hen Night Accessories) of the online Virgin Restoration Kits discussed here recommend the use of vaginal tightening creams as a supplement.[61]

Postoperative Care

I recommend employing traditional standards of icing for the first 24 to 48 hours, as tolerated, and standard analgesic regimens. Wound care consists of gentle irrigation after urination and patting after defecation. Patients are encouraged to take showers, but they should not bathe; sitz baths (cold is better than warm) are allowed for relief or cleansing; and patients should not use public pools, hot tubs, and saunas for 4 weeks.[63] Limited physical activity with no exercise for 4 weeks is advised. Patients are instructed not to use tampons. Light applications of ointment to sanitary pads or the use of nonadherent

Telfa pads to prevent sticking is suggested. One of the most important instructions is to not inspect the wounds (which may cause disruption). This will be done at the first postoperative visit, 4 weeks after surgery.

Rarely, a patient may be subjected to impending visual inspection for an intact hymen. In this case, sutures may be removed at the 3- to 4-week visit. However, sutures are usually completely absorbed in 6 to 8 weeks.

Evaluation of Results

Results are based on the outcome desired, which is usually bleeding during penetration. While practitioners may judge the success of the procedure by achieving an intact repair, this is less important to patients who assess the outcome by bleeding or tightness and pain with "first" coitus. I seek the patient satisfaction demonstrated in the following cellular text message a patient sent to me the day after her marriage. (The spelling and punctuation have not been corrected.) "Everthin is ok if u know what I mean [bleeding occurred] dnt text back ttyl [talk to you later] I'm with my hubby tell everyone thanks." This woman was told she would be immediately divorced and had concerns for bodily harm if she did not bleed as verification of her virginity.

Results and Outcomes

The results of these repairs are extremely difficult to assess because of a lack of follow-up; therefore "success" rates vary. In a report of 20 patients who underwent surgical adhesion of hymenal fragments, of whom 10 followed up, Longmans et al[30] stated that all 10 had a satisfactory outcome. Ou et al[60] performed Longman's technique in 2 patients and reported a need for a repeat procedure in both (100% failure) but cited that all 6 patients who underwent cerclage repair reported "no regrets." van Moorst et al[1] showed that of 24 patients, 19 returned for follow-up, only 2 (11%) bled with penetration, and 17 (89%) did not. However, despite the number of patients who did not bleed, 13 of 19 (68%) stated that they would have had the procedure again, and all of the 19 surgical patients said they had no regrets about having the procedure.

In my experience, in six of seven patients (undergoing the described procedure) contacted electronically or examined physically the repair was deemed successful. Success was defined as two or three intact adhesions at the 1-month postoperative visit or bleeding during coitus. One of seven patients was examined 4 weeks after surgery; one of three adhesions had healed. This patient was treated with a 5-0 chromic transluminal catgut suture 5 days before her marriage to ensure bleeding; bleeding on consummation was later confirmed.

Problems and Complications

Little is written about problems and complications of hymenoplasty other than the outcomes discussed previously and the social, religious, cultural, and ethical implications already reviewed. Most authors report that complications are minor; however, some mention, without documentation, the risks of "distortion, overvigorous repair with secondary dyspareunia or inhibition of penetration, separations of incisions, additional defects on the hymenal ring after surgery; deception of the male partner, and perpetuation of social injustice toward women"[59]; failure to bleed; and serious medical complications.[3,5,13] We know that if surgery is limited to the hymen, hymenal injuries tend to heal rapidly and leave no evidence of a previous injury, as demonstrated in a study of adolescent girls.[32]

Hymenoplasty is an interesting procedure in that the most common complication is wound dehiscence, which is essentially a natural state of the hymen on injury. In the series of cases discussed by Longmans et al,[30] Ou et al,[60] and van Moorst et al,[1] failure to bleed and repair breakdown were the only complications reported.[1,30,60] They did not report on the cultural consequences of those who did not bleed, but the limited follow-up of the van Moorst study (probably the least biased) showed that 19 of 24 women who underwent the procedure had no regrets.

References

1. van Moorst BR, van Lunsen RH, van Dijken DK, et al. Backgrounds of women applying for hymen reconstruction, the effects of counselling on myths and misunderstandings about virginity, and the results of hymen reconstruction. Eur J Contracept Reprod Health Care 17:93, 2012.
2. World Health Organization (WHO). Female genital mutilation: an overview. Geneva, Switzerland: World Health Organization, 1998. Available at *http://apps.who.int/iris/bitstream/ 10665/42042/1/9241561912_eng.pdf.*
3. O'Connor M. Reconstructing the hymen: mutilation or restoration? J Law Med 16:161, 2008.
4. Webb E. Cultural complexities should not be ignored. BMJ 316:462, 1998.
5. Cook RJ, Dickens BM. Hymen reconstruction: ethical and legal issues. Int J Gynecol Obstet 107:266, 2009.
6. Essén B, Blomkvist A, Helström L, et al. The experience and responses of Swedish health professionals to patients requesting virginity restoration (hymen repair). Reprod Health Matters 18:38, 2010.
7. Dobbeleir J, Landuyt K, Monstrey S. Aesthetic surgery of the female genitalia. Semin Plast Surg 25:130, 2011.
8. El Hennawy M. Hymenoplasty. Available at *http://www.powershow.com/view/3b58f5- MjAzZ/Hymenoplasty_Dr_Muhammad_El_Hennawy_Ob_gyn_specialist_Rass_powerpoint_ppt_ presentation.*
9. Kandela P. Egypt's trade in hymen repair. Lancet 347:1615, 1996.
10. Usta I. Hymenorrhaphy: what happens behind the gynaecologist's closed door? J Med Ethics 26:217, 2000.
11. Awwad J, Nassar A, Usta I, et al. Attitudes of Lebanese University students towards surgical hymen reconstruction. Arch Sex Behav 42:1627, 2013.

12. Eşsizoğlu A, Yasan A, Yildirim AE, et al. Double standard for traditional value of virginity and premarital sexuality in Turkey: a university student's case. J Womens Health 51:136, 2011.
13. Roberts H. Reconstructing virginity in Guatemala. Lancet 367:1227, 2006.
14. Paterson-Brown S. Commentary: education about the hymen is needed. BMJ 316:461, 1998.
15. Ahmadi A. Ethical issues in hymenoplasty: views from Tehran's physicians. J Med Ethics 40:429, 2014.
16. Philadelphoff-Puren N. Exhibiting the hymen: the blank page between law and literature. Stud Law Polit Soc 34:33, 2004.
17. Gürsoy E, Vural G. Nurses' and midwives' views on approaches to hymen examination. Nurs Ethics 10:485, 2003.
18. Raveenthiran V. Surgery of the hymen: from myth to modernization. Indian J Surg 71:224, 2009.
19. Cook S. The Islamic Garden. The myth of the hymen continues. Available at *http://www.islamicgarden.com/mythhymen.html.*
20. Committee on Gynecologic Practice, American College of Obstetricians and Gynecologists. ACOG Committee Opinion No. 378: Vaginal "rejuvenation" and cosmetic vaginal procedures. Obstet Gynecol 110:737, 2007.
21. Royal College of Obstetricians and Gynaecologists. Statement number 6: Hymenoplasty and Labial Surgery. London: Royal College of Gynaecologists, 2009.
22. Goodman MP, Bachmann G, Johnson C, et al. Is elective vulvar plastic surgery ever warranted, and what screening should be conducted preoperatively? J Sex Med 4:269, 2007.
23. Friedman RL. Surgery is not what it seems. BMJ 316:462, 1998.
24. Kopelman LM. Make her a virgin again: when medical disputes about minors are cultural clashes. J Med Philos 39:8, 2014.
25. Earp BD. Hymen 'restoration' in cultures of oppression: how can physicians promote individual patient welfare without becoming complicit in the perpetuation of unjust social norms? J Med Ethics 40:431, 2014.
26. Wild V, Neuhaus Bühler R, Poulin H, et al. [Requests for online consultations on the operative reconstruction of the hymen—data from the university hospital Zurich and the children's hospital Zurich] Praxis (Bern 1994) 99:475, 2010.
27. Raphael DD. Commentary: the ethical issue is deceit. BMJ 316:461, 1998.
28. Amy JJ. Certificates of virginity and reconstruction of the hymen. Eur J Contracept Reprod Health Care 13:111, 2008.
29. Helgesson G, Lynöe N. Should physicians fake diagnoses to help their patients? J Med Ethics 34:133, 2008.
30. Longmans A, Verhoeff A, Raap RB, et al. Should doctors reconstruct the vaginal introitus of adolescent girls to mimic the virginal state? Who wants the procedure and why? BMJ 316:459, 1998.
31. Hobday AJ, Haury L, Dayton PK. Function of the human hymen. Med Hypotheses 49:171, 1997.
32. McCann J, Miyamoto S, Boyle C, et al. Healing of hymenal injuries in prepubertal and adolescent girls: a descriptive study. Pediatrics 119:1094, 2007.
33. Curtis E, San Lazaro C. Appearance of the hymen in adolescents is not well documented. BMJ 318:605, 1999.
34. Edgardh K, Ormstad K. The adolescent hymen. J Reprod Med 47:710, 2002.
35. Mor N, Merlob P, Reisner SH. Types of hymen in the newborn infant. Eur J Obstet Gynecol Reprod Biol 22:225, 1986.
36. Gardner JJ. Descriptive study of genital variation in healthy, nonabused premenarchal girls. J Pediatr 120:251, 1992.
37. Berenson AB, Heger AH, Hayes JM, et al. Appearance of the hymen in prepubertal girls. Pediatrics 89:387, 1992.
38. Berenson A, Heger A, Andrews S. Appearance of the hymen in newborns. Pediatrics 87:458, 1991.
39. Berenson AB. Appearance of the hymen at birth and one year of age: a longitudinal study. Pediatrics 91:820, 1993.
40. Berenson AB. A longitudinal study of hymenal morphology in the first 3 years of life. Pediatrics 95:490, 1993.

41. Heger AH, Ticson L, Guerra L, et al. Appearance of the genitalia in girls selected for nonabuse: review of hymenal morphology and nonspecific findings. J Pediatr Adolesc Gynecol 15:27, 2002

42. Goodyear-Smith FA, Laidlaw TM. What is an 'intact' hymen? A critique of the literature. Med Sci Law 38:289, 1998.

43. Berenson AB, Chacko MR, Wiemann CM, et al. Use of hymenal measurements in the diagnosis of previous penetration. Pediatrics 109:228, 2002.

44. Stewart ST. Hymenal characteristics in girls with and without a history of sexual abuse. J Child Sex Abus 20:521, 2011.

45. Loeber O. Over het zwaard en de schede; bloedverlies en pijn bij de eerste coïtus. Een onderzoek bij vrouwen uit diverse culturen. Tijdschr Seks 32:129, 2008.

46. Prakash V. Hymenoplasty—how to do. Indian J Surg 71:221, 2009.

47. Emans SJ, Woods ER, Allred EN, et al. Hymenal findings in adolescent women: the impact of tampon use and consensual sexual activity. J Pediatr 125:153, 1994.

48. Cunningham FG, MacDonald PC, Gant NF, et al. Anatomy of the reproductive tract. In Cunningham FG, MacDonald PC, Gant NF, et al, eds. Williams Obstetrics, ed 20. Norwalk, CT: Appleton & Lange, 1997.

49. Rogers DJ, Stark M. The hymen is not necessarily torn after sexual intercourse. BMJ 317:414, 1998.

50. Goodyear-Smith FA, Laidlaw TM. Can tampon-use cause hymen changes in girls who have not had sexual intercourse? A review of the literature. Forensic Sci Int 94:147, 1998.

51. Adams JA, Botash AS, Kellogg N. Differences in hymenal morphology between adolescent girls with and without a history of consensual sexual intercourse. Arch Pediatr Adolesc Med 158:280, 2004.

52. Karaşahin KE, Alanbay I, Ercan CM, et al. Comment on a cerclage method for hymenoplasty. Taiwan J Obstet Gynecol 48:203, 2008.

53. Heppenstall-Heger A, McConnell G, Ticson L, et al. Healing patterns in anogenital injuries: a longitudinal study of injuries associated with sexual abuse, accidental injuries, or genital surgery in the preadolescent child. Pediatrics 112:829, 2003.

54. Cartwright R, Cardozo L. Cosmetic vulvovaginal surgery. Obstetrics, Gynaecol Reprod Med 18:285, 2008.

55. Duggal NL, Mercado C, Daniels K, et al. Antibiotic prophylaxis for prevention of postpartum perineal wound complications: a randomized controlled trial. Obstet Gynecol 111:1268, 2008.

56. Buppasiri P, Lumbiganon P, Thinkhamrop J, et al. Antibiotic prophylaxis for third- and fourth-degree perineal tear during vaginal birth. Cochrane Database Syst Rev 11:CD005125, 2010.

57. Renganathan A, Cartwright R, Cardozo L. Gynecological cosmetic surgery. Exp Rev Obstet Gynecol 4:101, 2009.

58. Tschudin S, Schuster S, Dumont dos Santos D, et al. Restoration of virginity: women's demand and health care providers' response in Switzerland. J Sex Med 10:2334, 2013.

59. Goodman MP. Female genital cosmetic and plastic surgery: a review. J Sex Med 8:1813, 2011.

60. Ou MC, Lin CC, Pang CC, et al. A cerclage method for hymenoplasty. Taiwan J Obstet Gynecol 47:355, 2008.

61. pbw. Menfolk behold the monster you created: wedding night survival kit for fake virgins. Available at *http://peacebenwilliams.com/menfolk-behold-the-monster-you-created-wedding-night-survival-kit-for-fake-virgins-see-photo/.*

62. pbw. Hymen Shop. Available at *http://www.hymenshop.com.*

63. Ramler D, Roberts J. A comparison of cold and warm sitz baths for relief of postpartum perineal pain. J Obstet Gynecol Neonatal Nurs 15:471, 1986.

CHAPTER 13

Auxiliary Procedures

Clara Santos, Red Alinsod

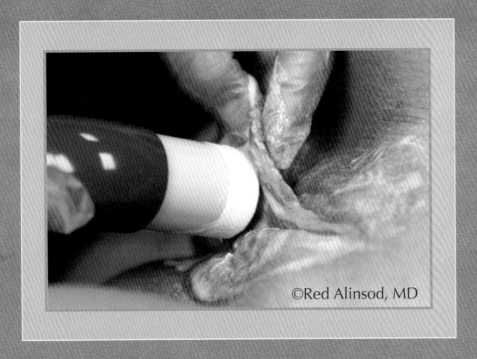

©Red Alinsod, MD

VULVAR LIGHTENING TECHNIQUES

Clara Santos

Key Points

- *Vulvar hyperpigmentation is caused by an increased concentration of melanin, which can occur in response to certain medical conditions, medications, and physical irritation. It can affect self-confidence and also sexual health.*

- *Treatments include the application of various acids that lighten and soften the affected area, lightening peels to resurface the skin, and fractional CO_2 lasers.*

Aesthetics is the set of principles that govern the ideas of beauty and artistic taste. It involves the perception and judgment of what is beautiful and the emotions that beauty provokes.

Today's selfie-sensitive patients are more than ever seeking physical perfection rather than only improvement. As women become more comfortable with the idea of elective procedures designed to enhance their appearance and self-confidence, it is not surprising that they may wish to alter, "rejuvenate," or reconstruct even more intimate areas of their bodies.[1]

Causes of Vulvar Hyperpigmentation

Skin color is formed by a combination of the pigments carotene, hemoglobin, and melanin. The main cause of vulvar hyperpigmentation is the production of melanin. Everyone has the same number of melanin-producing cells (melanocytes), regardless of ethnicity; however, the amount of melanin produced and how it is distributed will differ from person to person.

Benign pigmented hyperpigmentation of the vulva can occur in patients with dermatologic conditions such as lentigines, melanosis, postinflammatory hyperpigmentation, seborrheic keratoses, acanthosis nigricans, lentigo simplex, warts, lichen planus, discoid lupus erythematosus, and psoriasis. Systemic conditions such as Cushing disease and Addison disease can contribute to vulvar hyperpigmentation.[2]

Malignant pigmented lesions include some cases of vulvar intraepithelial neoplasia and melanoma.[3] A biopsy is always recommended when a diagnosis cannot be made with certainty after clinical examination and dermatoscopy.

Less commonly, drugs such as psoralens, bergamot, arsenic, and cytostatics can cause hyperpigmentation. Endocrine pathologic states such as kwashiorkor and adrenocorticotropic hormone excess, as well as endocrine physiologic states like pregnancy, can stimulate darkening of the genital area. In these conditions, patients' skin color response is mostly associated with pigments from hemoglobin and carotenes.

Most common causes of vulvar hyperpigmentation are physical in origin: waxing treatments for hair removal and the wearing of G-string undergarments and tight clothing or swimsuits. These practices result in excessive rubbing against the skin, which causes irritation and darkness of the vulvar-inguinal and perianal areas. This darkened skin may embarrass patients and affect their self-esteem.

Ideal Vulvar Aesthetics

Pigmented lesions of the genital mucosa are more frequent in women than in men.[4] Some women may seek vulvar or vaginal treatments either for purely cosmetic enhancements or for functional improvements. One of the most common reasons for a cosmetic consultation is vulvar hyperpigmentation. Even in the absence of functional concerns, vulvar hyperpigmentation causes many women to have poor self-confidence, which may lead to sexual impairment.

Chemical Agents Used for Vulvar Lightening

Lactic Acid

Lactic acid belongs to the alpha-hydroxy acid group and is a gentle acid commonly used in many skin care products. It is naturally occurring and present in sour or fermented milk. Lactic acid improves skin hydration, coloration, and quality. This chemical agent has moisturizing, exfoliating, and skin-lightening properties. As a moisturizer, lactic acid improves the skin hydration level by creating a barrier to hold moisture inside skin cells. The exfoliation property of lactic acid gently removes dead skin cells. After the skin scales, the new, younger skin looks softer and smoother. For skin lightening, the use of low concentrations of lactic acid for multiple cell cycles evens the skin tone.

Azelaic Acid

Azelaic acid is produced by *Malassezia furfur,* which is a yeast that lives on normal skin. Its main chemical properties are antimicrobial and keratolytic, and it also removes free radicals. Originally, azelaic acid was used to treat rosacea and grade I and II acne. With regard to hyperpigmentation, azelaic acid is used for its skin-lightening properties and as a tyrosinase inhibitor to reduce melanin synthesis. It also has antioxidant and bactericidal properties.

Mandelic Acid

Mandelic acid is extracted from bitter almonds. It has exfoliative properties, and it gently adheres to the skin to peel away dead skin cells. Like glycolic acid and lactic acid, mandelic acid is an alpha-hydroxy acid. The bigger size of its molecule (as compared with glycolic acid and lactic acid) favors less penetration into the skin and thus less irritation. It also has bactericidal and moisturizing properties.

Lightening Techniques

Chemical Peel

A chemical peel is an older but nonetheless excellent technique for resurfacing the skin. After the skin peels, the new skin surface is lighter and smoother. Chemical peel treatment of the external genital skin is more difficult because of the sensitivity of the tissue in this area. Another challenge is in determining the extent of the area to treat, because the excess pigmentation may extend beyond the labia majora skin and affect the inner groin region. Because of the natural folds of the skin of the groin area rubbing with movement and against clothing, the skin in this area can be easily damaged. However, some chemical peel agents and formulations have been used in these areas with good results, including formulations combining phytic, retinoic, and azelaic acid in low concentrations.

G-Peel

The G-Peel is a compound formulation mainly used for genital lightening. The agents' combination works by reducing the hyperpigmentation without creating skin damage.

G-Peel treatments involve eight office visits. Patients should undergo trichotomy the day before each visit. Right before the peel, the affected area should be cleansed with the use of a pH neutral soap. Protecting the mucosa with gauze afterward is important. The solution is applied to the darkened areas of the vulva and the labia majora using a disposable brush, and it is left on for 15 to 20 minutes. The peel solution is removed with water. The skin usually appears to be calm, and patients should have no discomfort. If a patient reports any irritation during the procedure, the peel solution should be removed immediately. For patients with no concerns, the peel is repeated every 15 days for 2 months until the desired results are achieved.

Home care after this procedure lasts for 2 months and is easy to perform. For cleansing, patients should use gentle soap products that contain lactobacilli, which work to restore the natural vaginal pH. The ideal active ingredients for these products include chamomile, aloe vera, and calendula. Patients should avoid soaps that contain acid and scrubbing soaps. Patients should apply maintenance cream twice daily; this cream contains low concentrations of lightening agents such as vitamin C, phytic acid, and kojic acid as its main ingredients.

Fractional CO$_2$ Laser

Fractional lasers have been used for many dermatologic, gynecologic, and cosmetic procedures (see Chapter 17). A fractional CO$_2$ laser treats only a specific column of skin and thus leaves the surrounding tissue intact. This type of laser can be used for the treatment of vulvar pigmentation in selected patients with Fitzpatrick skin types I to III, because darker skin is prone to rebound hyperpigmentation.

Safety Precautions

To treat the genital skin, the use of peel agents and lasers requires care to prevent burning the skin and postinflammatory hyperpigmentation or hypopigmentation.

Treatment should be discontinued if patients develop any of the following:
- Redness
- Scaling
- Itching
- Burning

The session should be postponed until the skin is normal again if any such sensitivity develops.

Results

Patient examples of auxiliary procedures are shown in Figs. 13-1 and 13-2.

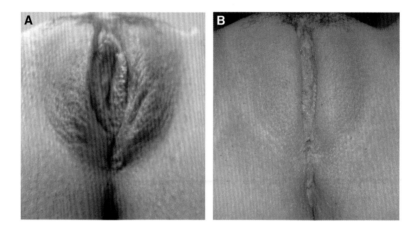

Fig. 13-1   A, This 32-year-old patient is shown before treatment. She had hyperpigmentation and lack of volume of her labia majora. **B,** After treatment. Hyaluronic acid filler was injected in her labia majora (5 cc on each side), and a G-Peel bleaching treatment was performed on the hyperpigmented areas.

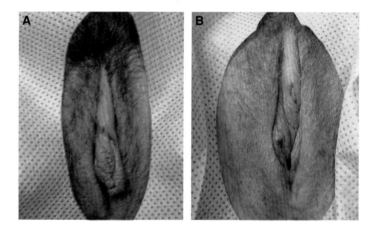

Fig. 13-2   A, This 58-year-old patient is shown before treatment. She had hyperpigmentation and post-menopausal volume loss in her labia majora. **B,** After treatment. Hyaluronic acid filler was injected in her labia majora (4 cc each side), and a G-Peel bleaching treatment was performed on the hyperpigmented areas.

Conclusion

In the presence of vulvar hyperpigmentation, lesions and certain medical conditions must be excluded, either through clinical diagnosis, dermatoscopy, or biopsy. The next step will be to bleach the vulvar skin to treat the hyperpigmentation. Appropriate care, peels, and lasers have definitely contributed to the beneficial results achieved, which have encouraged more patients to seek these types of treatments. As these techniques become more popular, more patients will benefit from them as ways to enhance their confidence and self-esteem.

DERMOELECTROPORATION FOR VULVOVAGINAL LIGHTENING

Red Alinsod

Key Points

- Dermoelectroporation® transiently lowers skin resistance and opens water channels to allow macromolecules to be transported through the skin.

- Ascorbic acid penetration of skin is very limited.

- Macromolecules such as BV-OSC (tetrahexyldecyl ascorbate) act as bioavailable antioxidants and whitening agents that can be used for vulvovaginal lightening.

- Vulvovaginal lightening can be achieved safely with Dermoelectroporation, but effects must be maintained with periodic treatments.

- Other macromolecules (such as collagen and hyaluronic acid) can be used with Dermoelectroporation to achieve a youthful appearance of the skin.

Electroporation: A Technology Used in Gene Therapy

Electroporation is a medical therapeutic method used for delivering life-saving drugs and beneficial genes directly into human cells. Three decades ago researchers discovered that briefly applying an electric field to a living cell causes a transient permeability in the cell's outer membrane.[5] This permeation is manifested by the appearance of pores across the membrane. After the field is discontinued, the pores close within 30 minutes without significant damage to the exposed cells and with the therapeutic molecules trapped inside the target cells. The phenomenon is known as *electroporation,* from the words *electric* and *pore.* Electroporation is now common in cancer therapy and as a DNA delivery method in gene therapy and DNA vaccination.

Short, high-voltage pulses can have dramatic and reversible effects on the skin's electrical properties. During a pulse, skin resistance drops as much as three orders of magnitude within microseconds. This alteration in skin resistance is either completely or partially reversible within minutes or longer. At relatively low voltages (less than 30 V), this drop in skin resistance can be attributed to electroporation of the appendages (for example, sweat glands and hair follicles). This effect allows targeted and specific aesthetic goals to be reached, such as vulvar and anal lightening.

For transdermal electroporation, the objective is to obtain a homogeneous distribution of an effective field. For the topical delivery of active agents through the skin, containing the electric field to a shallow skin surface layer is desirable so that the underlying nerves and muscles are not subjected to a strong electrical stimulation. After breakdown of the stratum corneum by electroporation, the depth of the electric field is related to the electrode spacing. A narrow spacing of multiple electrodes will confine the field to a surface region and therefore is a preferred configuration that can allow targeted lightening effects to a specific region such as the vulvovaginal area.

For human medical and nonmedical cosmetic applications, efficacy and sensation are very important criteria. The results of studies show that at least four factors influence these important considerations: formulation and its corresponding pH value, electrode design, electrical parameters, and skin site.[5] For cosmeceuticals, the preferred formulation is stable and has a neutral pH. The stability of the formulation determines the period of time over which the substrate (for example, collagen) will be active in the skin.

Dermoelectroporation: A No-Needle Transdermal Substance Delivery Method

Dermoelectroporation—as the name suggests—refers to the dermatology derivative of electroporation, optimized for the delivery of ionic substrates into the dermis and hypodermis. Dermoelectroporation is the patented technology developed in Florence, Italy, many years ago by Mattioli Engineering and clinically researched and tested at Siena University.[5] A zero-average current allows the use of all types of ionic solutions (not only those approved for iontophoresis) because of the absence of electrolytic reactions at the electrodes. Clinical trials have demonstrated the possibility to obtain, for the first time ever, transdermal delivery of macromolecules (1,000,000 Dalton or more) like collagen, hyaluronates, elastin, vitamin C, kojic acid, and hydroquinone; this suggests potential applications of new types of substances impossible to deliver by classical iontophoresis, which is restricted to lower-weight molecules.

Dermoelectroporation Studies

Since Bacchi[5] at Siena University, Italy, reported on the initial clinical trials using Dermoelectroporation, more than 4000 published scientific reports have been presented, discussing the results and possibilities of the method.

Biologically active drugs and macromolecules such as peptide drugs, proteins, oligo-nucleotides, and glycosaminoglycans are characterized by short biological half-lives and scarce bioavailability. Such characteristics make these difficult to employ for therapeutic strategies other than parenteral ones, which often are only practicable in hospitals. In a case study, the authors used a Dermoelectroporation technique, which involved the Transderm® Ionto System® (Mattioli Engineering) or Collagenizer® device (Vitality Concepts)[6] (see Fig. 13-3). Moreover, the transdermal delivery of biologically active molecules in vivo was analyzed. The advantage of using controlled electric pulses versus direct current application showed a significant reduction in the degradation of the molecules to be transdermally delivered.

Three sections were investigated:
    Section 1. Microscopic analysis of skin tissue after the application of the electric field
    Section 2. Qualitative analysis of transdermal delivery of a protein macromolecule
       (collagen type 1)
    Section 3. Quantitative analysis of transdermal delivery of lidocaine

The study showed that Dermoelectroporation can be used for transdermal delivery of biologically active molecules, in this case, a large protein macromolecule (collagen type 1) and a general anesthetic molecule (lidocaine).

This protocol is suitable for patients with the effects of acne or the initial stages of skin aging without tissue yield, and for the upkeep of aesthetic surgery results in facial and corporeal areas. The protocol consists first of a surface dermabrasion performed with corundum crystals to remove the corneum layer and for vascularization. Immediately afterward, active substances are introduced using the Dermoelectroporation method—a new, one-burst delivery method consisting of a controlled delivery of electrical pulses that causes "intercellular gates" in the dermis cells, thereby allowing the transdermal passage of molecules.[7] A vibration feature completes the Dermoelectroporation process by stimulating the Merkel corpuscles for greater connective restructuring of the tissue itself.

Dermoelectroporation Treatment

During the early 1970s, a group of American dermatologists discovered a change in polarization of the cellular membrane that could be used to promote a kind of cellular "pulsation" by applying an intense electric impulse for a short time at an adequate wavelength.[8] After the initial shock, the polarity conveyed was slowly reversed, production of electrolysis was avoided, and intercellular channels opened, through which substances could pass. This method was coined "electroporation treatment" and was used, with special techniques, in the transdermal treatment of melanoma.

To achieve an electroporation effect, a transmembrane voltage (0.5 to 1.5 V) is generated through a controlled sequence of electrical pulse delivery. These pulses cause the lipid components in the cellular membrane to form water-based channels and to open skin pores. These alterations give the membranes greater permeability to a large variety of hydrophilic molecules that otherwise could not enter the skin. Once these channels are formed, they remain open for a relatively long time, about several seconds. Dermoelectroporation follows the same rules. However, it does not injure cells or alter the membrane. In contrast to electroporation, Dermoelectroporation delivers lower-voltage electrical pulses having a suitable waveform, thus preventing an electrolysis effect while allowing intracellular channels to open and the active substance to penetrate into the skin.

The Dermoelectroporation device uses a pulsed delivery circuitry that allows macromolecules (for example, collagen, hyaluronic acid, elastin, vitamin C, kojic acid, and lidocaine) to be transdermally delivered into the dermis.[9] This novel technology delivers bursts of pulses with inversed polarity, preventing electrolysis effects at the electrodes while fully retaining the transdermal delivery effect using low-powered voltages and low current. Patients have no discomfort, and no adverse effects occur.

Together with the delivery of a specific pulse train, a mechanical vibration of 50 to 100 Hz is applied, causing a gentle sinusoidal trend and a stimulation of the Merkel corpuscles. The vibration assists the treatment in two ways:

1. Anesthetic effect: The electrical pulse frequency is equal to or double the vibration frequency. This causes an analgesic effect as vibration overcomes the feeling of electrical pulses on the skin.
2. Vibration improves blood and lymphatic circulation; together with massage, this promotes penetration of the active substance into the dermis.

In 2003 the Nobel Prize in Chemistry was awarded jointly to Drs. Peter Agre[10] and Roderick MacKinnon.[11] Their studies on the structure and operation of ion channels proved early evidence for a possible use of one of the most fascinating characteristics of the human dermis: the "hydroelectrophores." These are the water-based channels between cells that open as a result of physical, vibratory, mechanical, chemical, and nervous effects in a very spontaneous way and in a manner that allows the "external world" to communicate with the "interior universe" of cells. These water-based gates could open about 1,000,000,000,000,000,000,000.00 times per day.

We think that Dermoelectroporation can externally activate hydroelectrophores to transdermally deliver molecules even larger than those used in experimental studies on rats at the University of Florence, Italy. In this study, unaltered molecules of fluorescent bovine type 1 collagen with a size of 0.8 μ were transdermally delivered and monitored successfully.

A recent study in the Philippines showed a decrease in the melanin index, indicating significant skin lightening, which may be attributed to the functional whitening ingredients of the substrate (vitamin C) (personal communication).[12] Researchers used a stable, bioavailable, and oil-soluble form of vitamin C (BV-OSC) known to inhibit melanogenesis, inhibit tyrosinase activity, and act as an antioxidant to protect skin from DNA injury and UV-induced cell damage. The penetration of ascorbic acid is limited and dose dependent, and BV-OSC has a much higher penetration rate to provide this effect. The treatment showed a cumulative effect; repeated applications in 1-week intervals over 6 weeks resulted in significantly reduced melanin levels and visible lightening of skin.

We conducted a pilot study in our center in which we treated patients' vulvovaginal area. We aimed to prove the successful transport and expected efficacy of the substrates (medical-grade vitamin C cream). We performed one session per week for 5 weeks and allowed several weeks to pass without further treatments. Treatment times were approximately 15 minutes, depending on the size of the area treated (Figs. 13-3 through 13-7). The substrates appeared to have a sustained effect for at least 4 weeks. One reason the substrates remained within the dermal layer was that they were not easily excreted from the skin, as compared with substrates in the viable layers of the epidermis. The lightening effects appeared to be sustainable with periodic treatments. Maintenance treatments once a month appeared to maintain the effects obtained after a series of 4 to 6 weekly treatments. Dermoelectroporation has been well accepted as comfortable and effective for vulvar and anal lightening without the use of harsh chemicals such as hydrogen peroxide. Studies with combinations of lightening agents are ongoing at our center.

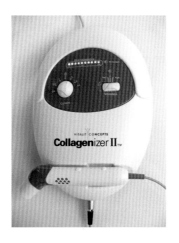

Fig. 13-3 The Collagenizer II device used for Dermoelectroporation.

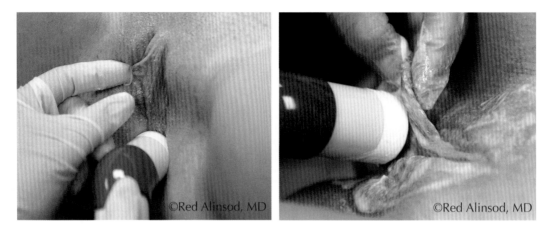

Fig. 13-4 Dermoelectroporation can be used both externally on the labial tissues and internally inside the vaginal canal. It can be performed to lighten skin tones and reduce pigmentation, as shown in these images. It can also be used with topical numbing agents to provide deep numbing effects before procedures such as labiaplasty and vaginoplasty.

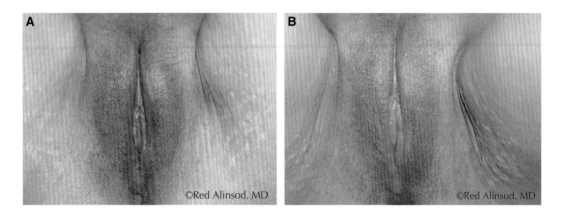

Fig. 13-5 **A,** This patient is shown before treatment. **B,** She has had five Dermoelectroporation sessions with BV-OSC.

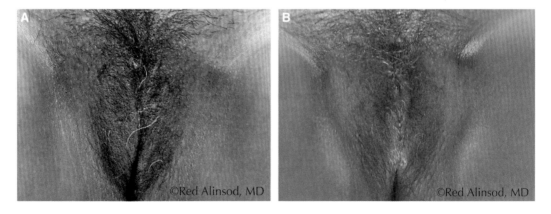

Fig. 13-6 **A,** This patient is shown before treatment. **B,** She has had five Dermoelectroporation sessions with BV-OSC.

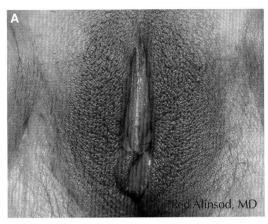
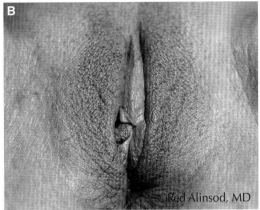

Fig. 13-7   **A,** This patient is shown before treatment. **B,** She has had five weekly treatments with Dermoelectroporation with BV-OSC and kojic acid.

Disclosure

Dr. Alinsod is a consultant for D-More Skin Care and Vitality Concepts, makers of Vitamin C Cream and the Collagenizer device.

References

1. Strauss DC, Thomas JM. What does the medical profession mean by "standards of care"? J Clin Oncology 27:192, 2009.
2. Haefner HK, Johnson TM, Rosamilia LL, et al. Pigmented lesions of the vulva. In Heller DS, Wallach RC, eds. Vulvar Disease: A Clinicopathological Approach. Boca Raton: CRC Press Taylor & Francis Group, 2007.
3. Rock B. Pigmented lesions of the vulva. Dermatol Clin 10:361, 1992.
4. Hengge UR, Meurer M. Pigmented lesions of the genital mucosa. Hautarzt 56:540, 2005.
5. Bacci PA. The role of dermoelectroporation. In Goldman MP, Bacci PA, Leibaschoff G, et al, eds. Cellulite: Pathophysiology and Treatment. New York: CRC Press Taylor & Francis Group, 2006.
6. Pacini S, Punzi T, Gulisano M, et al. Transdermal delivery of heparin using pulsed current iontophoresis. Pharm Res 23:14, 2006.
7. Pacini S, Perruzi B, Gulisano M. Qualitative and quantitative analysis of transdermic delivery of different biological molecules by iontophoresis. Ital J Anat Embryol 18(Suppl 2):127, 2003.
8. Prausnitz MR, Bose VG, Langer R, et al. Electroporation of mammalian skin: a mechanism to enhance transdermal drug delivery. Proc Natl Acad Sci U S A 90:10504, 1993.
9. Nestor M, Cazzaniga A. Pilot clinical study to evaluate the efficacy of the Transdermal Ionto device to minimize pain and discomfort associated with dermatological cosmetic procedures. Center for Cosmetic Enhancement, Aventura, Florida, 2005.
10. Agre P. Aquaporin water channels (Nobel Lecture). Agnew Chem Int Ed Engl 20:4278, 2004.
11. MacKinnon R. Nobel Lecture. Potassium channels and the atomic basis of selective ion conduction. Biosci Rep 24:75, 2004.
12. Chan GP, Chan H. The efficacy and safety of the Dermoelectroporation®-Collagenizer®II as a transdermal delivery device of large molecule substances for aesthetic improvement—an open pilot clinical trial (submitted for publication).

Part III
Advances

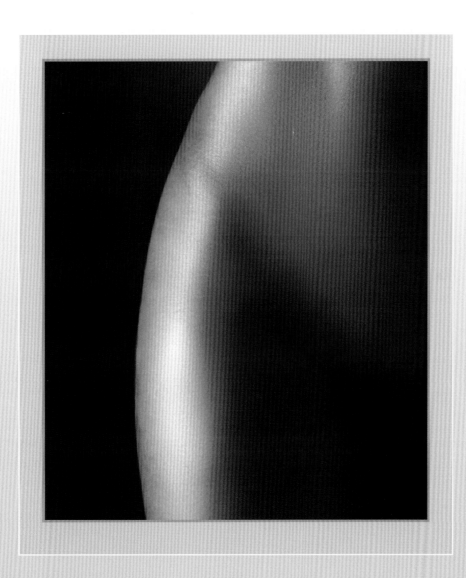

CHAPTER 14

Future Avenues and Advances

Colin C.M. Moore

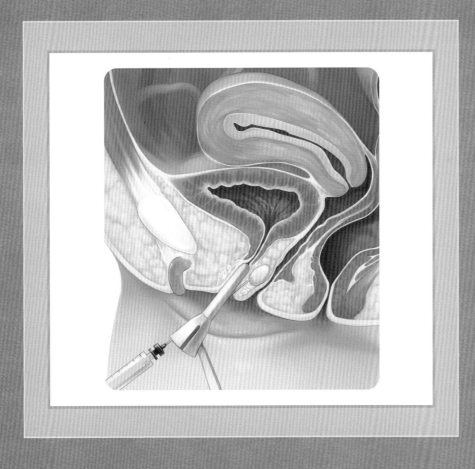

Key Points

- The G-spot is located below or inferior to the female urethra, approximately midway between the pubic bone and the cervix, and is responsible for vaginally activated orgasms.

- The precise anatomy of the G-spot is not completely understood.

- Vaginal laxity can be treated with vaginoplasty, which involves lifting the vaginal mucosa to tighten the sling muscles, removing excess vaginal lining, and reattaching the muscles.

- Vulvovaginal atrophy can be treated with vaginal estrogens, systemic estrogens, radiofrequency (RF), and laser therapies.

- Laser vaginal rejuvenation is a minimally invasive, temporary treatment that can be performed alone or after vaginoplasty.

- RF vaginal restoration promotes collagen formation and remodeling and is a temporary treatment; similar to laser rejuvenation, it may prove to be an effective treatment after vaginoplasty.

The G-Spot

History

Seldom in modern medicine, and particularly in sexology and sexual medicine, has there been so much reactivity as that related to the female orgasm in general and to the G-spot in particular. According to mythology, Tiresias, the son of a shepherd and a nymph, was punished by the goddess Hera for hitting a pair of copulating snakes and, in punishment, was turned into a woman. Later, Tiresias became embroiled in an argument between Zeus and Hera over who has more pleasure during sex: the man, as claimed by Hera, or the woman, as claimed by Zeus. As a woman who had once been a man, Tiresias was deemed to know the answer and replied, "of 10 parts, a man only enjoys one." Hera instantly struck Tiresias blind for his (or her) impiety and for revealing the secret of the female orgasm. This myth shows how, for whatever reason, the truth about female sexuality has largely been hidden, even since ancient times.[1]

In the twentieth century, modern Western culture had moved toward the belief that women were incapable of an intense orgasm, except by clitoral manipulation. This concept was reinforced by the work of Masters and Johnson,[2] whose research claimed that a woman's clitoris was the only source of female pleasure, even though many women had found that this was far from the truth.

This misguided notion persisted until 1950, when an article by the German gynecologist Ernst Gräfenberg[3] drew attention to his findings of a highly erotic area in the female urethra approximately midway between the pubic bone and the cervix. Drs. John Perry and Beverly Whipple[4] named this area of the urethra the Gräfenberg spot or the G-spot.

Whipple—co-author of *The G-Spot and Other Discoveries About Human Sexuality*[5]—claimed that the G-spot was overlooked by so many physicians during the first half of the nineteenth century for two reasons. First, the G-spot lies on the anterior wall of the vagina, which is an area that is not palpated during a normal vaginal examination. When physicians palpate this area in their patients, the patients have a sexual response. Second, doctors are trained not to sexually stimulate their patients. Whipple claimed that all gynecologists who palpated this area according to her and Dr. Perry's instructions found the erotic area. All members of this early group of physicians later reported back to Whipple's research group that they had subsequently found the erotic area of the urethra (G-spot) in every woman examined.

Orgasm Types

Women can have two kinds of orgasm. However, they are not strictly "clitoral" versus "vaginal," as some authors have reported. Rather, they are "clitorally activated" versus "vaginally activated." In their study on vaginally activated orgasms versus clitorally activated orgasms, Jannini et al[6] showed that orgasms resulting from direct clitoral stimulation have been reported to be sharp, bursting, short-lasting, superficial, and more localized, confined only to the pubic area.[7,8] By contrast, vaginally activated orgasms have been described as more diffuse, whole-body, radiating, psychologically more satisfying, and longer lasting.[6-8] It has been further shown that women who have both types of orgasm have even deeper, more powerful, blended orgasms resulting from contractions in both areas at once.

The most common orgasm (sometimes called a *clitorally activated orgasm*) also involves the vagina, because clitoral stimulation produces contractions of the pubococcygeal muscle supporting the pelvic floor, which is where vaginal contractions are felt. Orgasms that result from G-spot stimulation involve the vagina as well but cause contractions around the uterus, which is several inches above the pelvic floor, and may also involve the muscles of the lower part of the anterior abdominal wall.

Anatomy of the G-Spot

The anatomic structures that might provoke a vaginally activated orgasm, rather than a clitorally activated orgasm, have not been completely and unequivocally described. This is probably the result of major uncertainty regarding human gross anatomy (Fig. 14-1). After the publication of the book *The G-Spot and Other Discoveries About Human Sexuality*[5] in 1982, many scientists began the search for a specific, discrete organ or site within the anterior vaginal wall with a high nerve density that could explain the increased sensitivity of this region reported by many women.[9,10]

Recently, Gravina et al[11] demonstrated a direct correlation between the thickness of the urethrovaginal space, or G-spot, and vaginal orgasms. Zaviacic et al[12] affirmed that the urethrovaginal space is occupied by the female prostate. On the other hand, Crooks and Baur[13] reported that the G-spot consists of a system of glands (Skene glands) and ducts that surround the urethra. The female prostate has been considered as an afunctional,

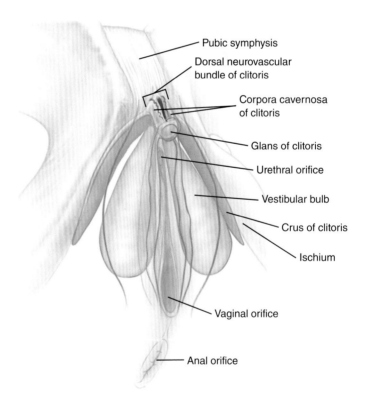

Fig. 14-1 Gross anatomy of the vaginal introital area of the vulva.

vestigial gland. Zaviacic and Albin[14] demonstrated that the prostate can be considered as another organ in both males and females, having a different size, weight, and function, yet the same qualitative parameters in both genders. Battaglia et al[15] studied a group of women by ultrasound and color Doppler examination. The urethrovaginal space and the clitoral body were scanned with high-resolution ultrasound using the color Doppler mode.

Gravina et al[11] examined the urethrovaginal space along a line drawn between the border of the smooth muscle, the mucosal-submucosal layer of the urethral wall, and the border of the vaginal wall and its lumen. The three-dimensional reconstruction of the urethrovaginal space had a glandlike aspect with small feeding vessels. Komisaruk et al[16] confirmed the presence of several different organs in this highly complex body region. They stated that this area may include the anterior vaginal wall, the urethra itself, the Skene glands (including the periurethral glands, also known as the *female prostate gland*), perhaps the other glands in this region (vestibular glands and Bartholin glands), the surrounding muscle and connective tissue, and possibly the crura of the clitoris. Gravina et al[11] demonstrated that women who reported vaginally activated orgasms had a larger distance between the urethra and the vaginal mucosa than women who reported having no vaginally activated orgasm, thereby suggesting a bigger and possibly more active cliterourethrovaginal complex (G-spot). This finding was confirmed by other researchers, who found that vaginally activated orgasms were associated not only with a thicker, but also with a longer urethrovaginal septum.[17]

In addition to the potentially important role of engorgement of the vascular erectile components of the cliterourethrovaginal complex during sexual arousal,[17] these tissues were located superficially below the mucosal layer of the vagina in a cadaveric autopsy study.[18] Based on this anatomic finding, subvaginal filling (as in G-spot augmentation), performed transvaginally is potentially incorrect. These findings suggest that the filler should be placed closer to the urethra than to the vaginal wall.

The clitoris is innervated mainly by the pudendal nerve (see Fig. 1-11), the vagina primarily by the pelvic nerves, and the cervix by the hypogastric, pelvic, and vagus nerves.[8] If several neural pathways are activated during cliterourethrovaginal complex stimulation (the pelvic, hypogastric, and vagus nerves), whereas only the pudendal nerve is directly stimulated during clitoral stimulation, this could at least partially explain perceptual differences between clitorally activated orgasms and vaginally activated orgasms.

In a recent study by anatomic dissection of fresh frozen cadavers, Ostrzenski[19] identified the G-spot as an elongated structure lying on the superodorsal perineal membrane at an

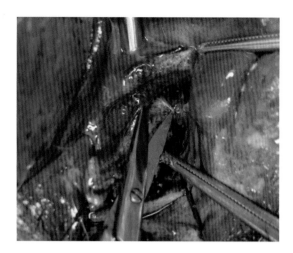

Fig. 14-2 The G-spot is seen as bluish, grapelike compositions between the supero-dorsal perineal membrane and the inferior pubocervical fascia and grossly resembling that cavernous tissue, which creates a 35-degree angle with the lateral urethra. The ropelike structure emerges from the tail that disappears into the adjacent tissue. The lower pole measures 3 mm and the upper pole 15 mm from the urethra. The G-spot's housing looked grossly like the fibroconnective tissues.

oblique angle of 35 degrees dorsal (that is, vaginalward) to the urethra, with the perineal-ward pole lying 3 mm from the urethra, the cervivalward pole 15 mm from the urethra, and the whole structure parallel to the urethra (Fig. 14-2).

Treatment

Patient History and Physical Examination

All women have a G-spot. Not all women have G-spot (cliterourethrovaginal complex) orgasms. The reason may be that the clitoris is superficial and easily stimulated, whereas the G-spot is hidden and more difficult to stimulate. Both women and men initially tend to concentrate on stimulation of the clitoris, especially during autostimulation; however, some women discover their G-spot during their immediate postpubertal years and learn to stimulate it. These women are more likely to have G-spot orgasms than those focused only on the clitoris. Therefore, when taking a patient's history, determining what kind of orgasm the patient has is essential. Patients who do not have vaginally activated (G-spot) orgasms need to be taught how to achieve these, because simply augmenting the G-spot will not guarantee that a patient will have G-spot orgasms (see Self-Discovery of the G-Spot).

A physical examination, apart from a standard general examination, requires a vaginal examination that includes locating the patient's G-spot. With the fingers gently inserted into the vagina about 5 to 6 cm past the introitus and beneath the pubic bone, pressure on the anterior vaginal wall roughly midway between the pubic bone and the cervix will initially cause a desire to micturate. After releasing and reapplying pressure, the patient will eventually report that this produces erotic and pleasing feelings. The examiner should stop at this point, record the depth of the G-spot in relation to a fixed anatomic landmark such as the urethral orifice, and continue to inform the patient verbally. The recorded depth of the G-spot will be useful later during G-spot augmentation.

Self-Discovery of the G-Spot

Nonvaginally activated patients must be taught how to stimulate their G-spot. They should have G-spot–induced orgasms before undergoing G-spot augmentation. This will help to ensure quality results. To do this, the patient helps me to find her G-spot (in the presence of my nurse). Once located, the exact site is recorded. The patient sits upright and is shown how and where to identify her own G-spot using her fingers. This can be difficult for some patients. In these cases, I take a G-spot vibrator and locate the spot for her. She then reinserts the vibrator herself and locates the site of the erotically centered spot on her anterior vaginal wall. If she has brought her own vibrator with her, we use it, and we mark the front edge of the vibrator to assist her with finding the correct depth when attempting this at home. Most patients learn the technique easily, although some require more than one session. I advise them to sit in front of a mirror at home with the thighs fully abducted and slightly flexed at the hips to expose the vaginal introitus. They should proceed as shown in my examination room. I think having a nurse chaperone (not a friend or family member) is critical. I wear gloves to clinically and psychologically emphasize as much as possible the nonpersonal nature of this highly intimate examination. About 35% of women are unable to convert to even mild G-spot orgasms. I refer these patients to a sex therapist, which is helpful in many cases (approximately 15%). Some are lost to follow-up, and some continue to have therapy.

Women Who Do Not Have G-Spot Orgasms

As part of the physical examination, once the physician has located the G-spot, the patient should be shown where it is by having her insert her fingers along the anterior vaginal wall until she feels the same sensation that the examiner was able to cause during the examination. The patient should be told to acquire a so-called G-spot vibrator, which is specially shaped to stimulate the anterior vaginal wall so that she can improve her G-spot sensations in the privacy of her own home. The patient's partner should also be taught to locate the position of the G-spot and to perform the "come hither" finger technique, which he can use to stimulate his partner's G-spot.

Women Who Have G-Spot Orgasms

Platelet-rich plasma and other methods of G-spot augmentation should be given *only* to women who have had G-spot orgasms, however inadequate. These techniques will *only* enhance the duration and intensity of G-Spot orgasms in these women. These methods, in my experience, will *not* induce G-spot orgasms in women who have not had G-spot orgasms.

Platelet-Rich Plasma

Platelet-rich plasma is a new addition to this area (see Chapter 15). Experience with its use is limited, and there are no peer-reviewed articles about its use. I have made no conclusions about this product based on my own limited experience using it for improving G-spot performance. In the small number of cases that I have performed, none has reported improved G-spot orgasms, and none has converted from not having G-spot orgasms to having them.

Transvaginal Versus Transurethral Augmentation of the G-Spot

Augmentation of the G-spot works on the basis that bulking the G-spot forward toward the vaginal lumen on the vaginal wall will bring it into greater contact with the vaginal contents and increase the likelihood of the patient having longer and more intense G-spot orgasms. Current techniques for transvaginally instilling material such as collagen or other nonpermanent fillers or various permanent fillers into the anterior wall of the vagina do not—on the basis of current anatomic knowledge[8,11,13,15]—make a great deal of sense to me. The G-Shot®, as demonstrated by its inventor, David Matlock, is given either just into the subvaginal mucosa (that is, between the G-spot and the vaginal mucosa) or into the G-spot in the urethrovaginal septum (that is, directly into the G-spot itself).

Because the bulk of the G-spot tissues lies closer to the vaginal wall than to the urethral wall in the urethrovaginal septum, it makes more sense to place the bulking material just under the musculature of the urethra at about its midpoint (Figs. 14-3 and 14-4) to push the G-spot structures caudally (toward the vaginal lumen) and bring these structures closer to intravaginal contents such as a penis or a finger to facilitate stimulation.

I achieve this by injecting 1.5 to 2.5 ml of Macroplastique® (Cogentix Medical) transurethrally using a Storz Viscous Fluid Injection Set (see Fig. 14-3). Macroplastique is placed just under the muscularis of the urethra, above the previously determined G-spot to cause the G-spot to bulge vaginalward. Alternatively, the Macroplastique Implantation Device can be used, which involves a blind procedure and requires that the G-spot be palpated transvaginally to make sure that the tip of the device is in the urethra at the correct position (see Fig. 14-4). The needle is inserted and injection is completed.

Macroplastique is medical-grade silicone that is thermogravimetric analysis (TGA)–approved for periurethral and periureteric injection for various urologic indications. It is permanent and does not migrate or lose any appreciable volume. Macroplastique lasts forever, and if it is inadvertently placed incorrectly, it is fairly easy to remove. By contrast, hyaluronic acid is temporary, lasting only 12 to 18 months; if it is combined with Botox, it may last 2 to 2½ years. It can be diminished by injecting hyaluronidase to dispel it, but 100% removal takes time. Allergy to hyaluronic acid occurs occasionally, whereas allergy to silicone has never been reported, to my knowledge.

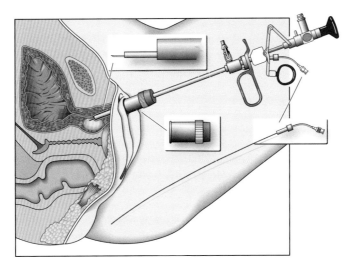

Fig. 14-3   Transurethral injection. A Storz Viscous Fluid Injection Set (Karl Storz GMBH & Co.) is used with the patient under light general anesthesia in the operating room. I think this is the most accurate technique, but it requires the operator to have some skill with urologic endoscopic instruments.

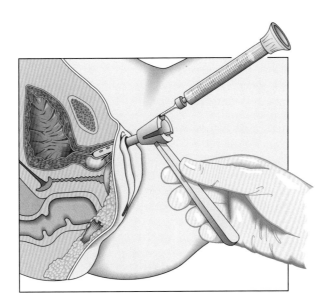

Fig. 14-4   The use of the Macroplastique Implantation Device. This technique is almost as accurate as the one shown in Fig. 14-3, especially when done with the patient under light general anesthesia. An advantage is that it can be employed in unsedated or unanesthetized patients using a local anesthetic-containing lubrication injected in the urethra in appropriately selected patients in the physician's office.

I have used either Macroplastique (silicon) or polyacrylamide gel (Aquamid, Contura) with equally good results.

The use of the temporary bulking agents can improve the local collagen content and collagen stimulation and increase blood flow if hyaluronic acid or Radiesse-type products and/or platelet-rich plasma is used. The increased localized blood flow can help to explain how these injections are working in some patients.

In my experience with 230 patients, some with clitoral-only and some with lesser-quality G-spot orgasms, this technique (Macroplastique or polyacrylamide gel delivered transurethrally) has produced excellent results with improved vaginal-activated orgasms in intensity and frequency. At this writing, 99% of the women in my practice who had lesser-quality G-spot orgasms before treatment have reported improved G-spot orgasms. The total number having good-quality G-spot orgasms is 189 (82% of the total series), and the total number having lesser-quality G-spot orgasms who converted to good-quality G-spot orgasms is 187, which is 99% of patients who qualified for injection therapy. Of those who did not have G-spot orgasms before treatment, only 65% were convertible with the method described previously in the section about women who do not have G-spot orgasms. However, 92.5% of my patients in this group have eventually had good-quality G-spot orgasms after treatment.

After the installation of either Macroplastique or polyacrylamide gel into the urethro-vaginal septum below the urethral musculature, urethral obstruction is a risk, at least temporarily. Therefore I place a 14 Fr Foley catheter into the bladder to splint the urethra so that the injected material will spread around the urethra and allow it to indent in a U-shaped manner. The catheter remains in place overnight and is removed the next morning. During this time, the Macroplastique or the polyacrylamide gel assumes the shape of the vaginal aspect of the catheter (pushing the G-spot structures vaginalward) and develops a periinjection material capsule (for example, as occurs around a breast implant); this contributes to its position stability and longevity. Patients are discharged after they are able to empty the bladder per the urethra.

In my experience, instilling 2.5 to 5 ml of either Macroplastique or polyacrylamide gel just below the urethral muscular wall in the midurethra usually achieves an excellent result.

Complications

The incidence of urinary obstruction in the early part of my series was 7 of 10. These patients were treated with the insertion of a urethral indwelling catheter for 12 hours and were discharged without any further problems. Thereafter, I started to routinely insert a urethral indwelling catheter immediately after injection, kept patients in the hospital overnight, and removed the catheter the next morning. After patients could pass urine per the urethra, they were discharged (usually later that morning).

Vaginoplasty

After childbirth, menopause, and the aging process, women may have stretched pelvic floor muscles and pelvic ligaments and skin changes that can alter the shape and function of the vagina internally and externally. These changes have been addressed with local hormone creams, lubricants, and surgery. They can also be treated with vaginoplasty (see Chapter 11), which involves tightening the sling muscles of the vagina by lifting the mucosa, removing excess vaginal lining, and reattaching the muscles, which have been tightened.

Before the climacteric period, the vagina is composed of thick layers of healthy cells, and estrogens encourage the growth and development of these cells. As a result, the vaginal epithelium remains multilayered, and its walls are supple and elastic.

The progressive reduction in circulating estrogens that occurs after the cessation of ovarian function during menopause induces tissue and metabolic changes that are most prominent in the genital tract because of its high sensitivity to variation in sex hormone levels.[20,21] Vulvovaginal atrophy is a progressive condition that is seen as involution of the vulvovaginal mucous membranes and tissues resulting from the menopausal drop in estrogen levels.[22,23]

The typical symptoms of vulvovaginal atrophy, which reflect these vulvovaginal morphofunctional changes, include vaginal dryness, itching, burning, irritation, dysuria, and dyspareunia. The vaginal walls appear thinner and less elastic with fewer rugations. The vaginal surface appears dry and friable and often bleeds after minimal trauma. The vulvar area, particularly the clitoris, becomes atrophic and more vulnerable.

Several therapeutic options are available for treating vulvovaginal atrophy symptoms. These include RF (see Chapter 16), platelet-rich plasma (see Chapter 15), hyaluronic acid filler, nonhormonal products, local vaginal therapy for persistent symptoms, and systemic hormonal replacement therapy. Lubricants have been shown to decrease vaginal irritation during sexual activity but do not provide a long-term solution. The major drawback to these approaches is the recurrence of symptoms once the particular treatment has been suspended. Furthermore, the treatment is effective usually only in the superficial layer of the vaginal wall.

Recently, demand has been increasing for a safe, long-term, therapeutic option that can effectively treat the deep layers of the vaginal mucosa, in addition to the epithelium. By applying the principles of regenerative and antiaging medicine to the vaginal mucosa, the use of fractional CO_2 laser may be extended to treat patients with vulvovaginal atrophy. As shown in other areas of the body,[24-27] fractional CO_2 laser induces the topical remodeling of connective tissue and the production of collagen and elastic fibers.

Laser Vaginal Rejuvenation

Based on the results obtained on the skin, Perino et al[28] applied fractional CO_2 laser treatment designed specifically for the vaginal mucosa. They showed that thermoablative fractional CO_2 laser is a safe, effective, and feasible option for the treatment of vulvovaginal atrophy symptoms in postmenopausal women.

In 2011 Gaspar et al[29] first demonstrated significant histologic improvement in vaginal biopsy specimens that had been treated with a fractional, microablative CO_2 laser in combination with platelet-rich plasma. They observed beneficial changes in the three layers of the vaginal wall in contrast to the changes induced by estrogens or other local therapies that only treat the epithelium.

Salvatore et al[30] recently published a pilot study on the use of fractional CO_2 laser to treat vulvovaginal atrophy in postmenopausal women. The results demonstrated a significant improvement in sexual function and overall satisfaction with sexual life. At the 12-week follow-up, approximately two thirds of the study patients showed signs of improvement. Vaginal dryness improved in 66% of patients, vaginal burning in 64%, vaginal itching in 67%, dyspareunia in 66%, and dysuria in 54% of the patients. Alinsod[31] performed a similar study at 12 weeks after three treatments with RF, which has shown near 100% improvement in dryness, burning, itching, and dyspareunia.

In a microscopic and ultrastructural study, Zerbinati et al[32] produced results that strongly support the hypothesis that the production of new collagen and ground substance components within the connective tissue and glycogen and acidic mucins within the epithelium can rebalance and restore vaginal mucosa from atrophy induced by the absence of ovarian estrogens, resulting in a highly significant improvement in clinical symptoms. This is true of laser treatment and RF. With RF, localized blood flow in the vagina is increased, resulting in increased vaginal transudate and improved sensitivity. In the study by Perino et al,[28] 91% of the patients who received CO_2 laser treatment declared that they were satisfied or very satisfied with the procedure, which corresponded to a considerable improvement in quality of life.

The duration of the vaginal changes induced by the laser application require clarification. Salvatore et al[30] confirmed that the effect on collagen remodeling, which they had preliminarily demonstrated in ex vivo vaginal specimens, was similar to what has been observed in vivo at the skin level. Currently, Mitch Goldman, in San Diego, is conducting a study to better understand how RF improves atrophic changes of the vulvovaginal region. From these studies, it seems that this relatively new therapeutic modality is primarily applicable for improving vaginal mucosal symptoms such as itching, dryness, burning, and dyspareunia in postmenopausal women.

This therapeutic modality may have some role in premenopausal females (see Chapter 16). However, it seems unlikely, because their main complaint is loss of tactile sensation in relation to intravaginal intercourse. This most commonly results from significant stretching of the pelvic floor muscles. At the time of writing, no evidence has shown that significant vaginal musculature tightening results from fractional CO_2 laser treatment. This is exactly analogous to what occurs in the face, where facial resurfacing with either erbium or old-style CO_2 lasers produces some tightening of the skin but nowhere near the changes that a surgical facelift is capable of producing. RF and lasers have different effects on tissues. RF is known to have healing effects on muscles and fascial tissues, and it is widely used in professional sports to help athletes heal torn or damaged muscle and fascial tissue faster. Anecdotal reports from RF-treated patients have documented more efficient, coordinated muscle function, because RF brings stretched fascia into closer proximity, allowing muscle to act as an organized unit. Patients interpret this coordinated action as stronger contraction of their muscles, although no muscle strength and function tests have been done.

An advantage of CO_2 laser vaginoplasty is its minimally invasive nature. It takes only 15 minutes and usually requires three treatments at monthly intervals. Patients can return to work later that same day or the next day. However, patients should not have sexual activity for up to 6 weeks after each treatment.

I think that eventually perimenopausal women who appear to have adequate vaginal mucosa and muscle laxity and whose only concern is decreased lubrication could benefit well from a combination of standard, surgical, posterior vaginoplasty and CO_2 laser vaginal rejuvenation about 6 weeks after the vaginoplasty surgery. Alternatively, surgeons can perform a surgical vaginoplasty, followed by an RF treatment immediately after the surgery, at the 6-week postoperative visit, and again a month later. This allows the development of a normal pH and a normal, moisturized vagina in the same healing timeframe as that needed for the surgery itself.

Radiofrequency Vaginal Rejuvenation

In 2010 Millheiser et al[33] reported on the first pilot study using nonsurgical RF treatment to subjectively improve vaginal tightness. In 2012 Sekiguchi et al,[34] from the Women's Clinic LUNA, in Japan, reported on a second series of 30 patients treated with RF for vaginal restoration. Alinsod[35] performed a pilot study in a similar manner with ThermiVa with 23 patients. He also conducted an unpublished, IRB-approved study that included more than 60 patients and that confirmed the results of the studies by Millheiser, Sekiguchi, and Alinsod.

Millheiser et al[33] and Sekiguchi et al[34] reported on women who had delivered vaginally and had a loss of vaginal sensation. The RF modality was applied only to the vaginal introitus and the tissues in the region of the periurethra and inner aspects of the labia minora. RF energy was chosen to treat these women, because it had a substantially safe history of use for noninvasive treatment of the lax skin of the face and neck[36,37] and for rhytids in the delicate tissue of the periorbital area,[38] based on the premise of thermal tissue remodeling rather than ablation. It relies on the concept that carefully controlled RF energy can be used to heat deeper, submucosal tissue, in conjunction with concomitant cryogen cooling to prevent superficial heat injury. The increased collagen formation appears to contribute to the mechanism of skin tightening over time,[39] with dermal collagen remodeling as a restorative process after exposure to RF thermal energy.

Millheiser et al[33] used sheep vagina as an animal model system and showed that temporal changes of collagen tissue remodeling in the sheep vagina reflected a possible mechanism to explain the human subjects' perceptions of increased vaginal tightness in the 1- to 6-month period after RF treatment. They further reported that over the period of 6 months after RF treatment, sexual function scores improved in their study sample of women, and their level of personal distress decreased significantly, with the Malay version of the Female Sexual Function Index scores higher than 15.

Sekiguchi et al[34] studied a series of 30 premenopausal Japanese women whose complaints were mainly of "vaginal emptiness" and a loss of physical/sexual sensation during vaginal intercourse. A single RF treatment was performed on each subject as an in-office procedure without prior sedation or analgesics. All 30 patients reported subjective improvements in vaginal integrity and increased sexual satisfaction.

In 2015 Alinsod[35] reported on a prospective study of 23 patients 26 to 58 years of age with vulvovaginal laxity treated with RF. Six of 23 subjects were lost to follow-up before each of the second and third treatments could be performed. They reported that they were highly satisfied with the results and did not need further treatment. The rest completed the second and third treatments. No burns, no blisters, or major complications occurred during or after treatments, which patients described as pleasant and very comfortable. Patients were able to resume all activity as normal, including sexual intercourse, immediately after each treatment. Furthermore, all patients with any kind of orgasmic dysfunction, including clitoral orgasmic dysfunction, reported dramatic improvement, for example, stronger, multiple, and/or more rapid achievement of orgasms with coordinated vaginal contracture during coitus. In a personal communication, Alinsod[40] has informed me that anorgasmia persisted in some patients, although they had improved sensitivity. Those who had previous reconstructive surgery with extensive anterior dissection did not respond well to RF treatments to improve sensitivity. Alinsod thought that this may have resulted from extensive dissection of the anterior compartment possibly disrupting the G-spot areas—a theory with which I agree, given the intricate microanatomy of the G-spot.

RF treatment of vaginal laxity after vaginal delivery in these three short series show very promising results. The reports are largely subjective, and a more objective measurement of outcomes is required. These results, however, seem to place RF in a similar place with vulvovaginal laxity as it enjoys with skin tightening in the face and periorbital areas. As with treatment in these areas, good results will likely depend on careful patient selection, and, when it is the only modality used, RF will prove to be of limited application. Based on the information currently available, RF does not seem to produce the kind of changes produced by surgical correction of the pelvic diaphragm, required for patients whose pelvic musculature has been damaged by childbirth. I think the application of RF *after* a surgical repair would be more appropriate, although Alinsod indicated that the shrinkage of prolapsed tissues by RF may, in selected patients, prevent the need for invasive surgery (personal communication, 2016). He therefore recommended RF before surgery.

References

1. Loraux N, ed. The Experiences of Tiresia. The Feminine and the Greek Man. Princeton, NJ: Princeton University Press, 1995.
2. Masters WH, Johnson EV, eds. Human Sexual Response. Boston: Little Brown, 1966.
3. Gräfenberg E. The role of the urethra in female orgasm. Int J Sexology 3:145, 1950.
4. Perry JD, Whipple B. Pelvic muscle strength of female ejaculators: evidence in support of a new theory of orgasm. J Sex Res 17:22, 1987.
5. Ladas AR, Whipple B, Perry JD, eds. The G-Spot and Other Discoveries About Human Sexuality. New York: Holt Rinehart and Winston, 1982.
6. Jannini EA, d'Amati G, Lenzi A. Histology and immunohistochemical studies of female genital tissue. In Goldstein I, Maston C, Davis S, et al, eds. Women's Sexual Function and Dysfunction Study, Diagnosis and Treatment. London: Taylor and Francis, 2006.
7. Komisaruk BR, Whipple B, Crawford A, et al. Brain activation during vagina cervical self-stimulation and orgasm in women with complete spinal cord injury: fMRI evidence of mediation of the vagus nerves. Brain Res 1024:77, 2004.
8. Komisaruk JB, Beyar-Flores C, Whipple B, eds. The Science of Orgasm. Baltimore: Johns Hopkins University Press, 2006.
9. Kilchevsky A, Vardi Y, Lowenstein L, et al. Is the female G-spot truly a distinct anatomic entity? J Sex Med 9:719, 2012.
10. Puppo V, Gruenwald I. Does the G-spot exist? A review of the current literature. Int Urogynecol J 23:1665, 2012.
11. Gravina GL, Brandetti F, Martini P, et al. Measurement of the thickness of the urethro-vaginal space in women with or without vaginal orgasm. J Sex Med 5:601, 2008.
12. Zaviacic M, Jakubovská V, Belosovic M, et al. Ultrastructure of the normal adult female prostate gland (Skene's gland). Anat Embryol (Berl) 201:51, 2000.
13. Crooks R, Baur K, eds. Our Sexuality, ed 7. Pacific Grove, CA: Brooks and Cole, 1999.
14. Zaviacic M, Albin RJ. The female prostate and prostatic-specific antigen. Immunohistochemical localization, implications of this prostate marker in women and reasons for using the term "prostate" in the human female. Histol Histopathol 15:131, 2000.
15. Battaglia C, Nappi RE, Mancini F, et al. PCOS and urethrovaginal space: 3-D volumetric and vascular analysis. J Sex Med 7:2755, 2010.
16. Komisaruk BR, Whipple B, Nauerzadeh S, et al, eds. The Orgasm Answer Guide, ed 2. Baltimore: Johns Hopkins University Press (in press).
17. Battaglia C, Nappi RE, Mancini F, et al. 3-D volumetric and vascular analysis of the urethrovaginal space in young women with and without vaginal orgasm. J Sex Med 7(4 Pt 1):1445, 2010.

18. Rees MA, O'Connell HE, Plenter RJ, et al. The suspensory ligament of the clitoris: connective tissue supports of the erectile tissues of the female urogenital region. Clin Anat 13:397, 2000.
19. Ostrzenski A. G-spot anatomy: a new discovery. J Sex Med 9:1355, 2012.
20. Sturdee DW, Panay N; International Menopause Society Writing Group. Recommendations for the management of postmenopausal vaginal atrophy. Climacteric 13:509, 2010.
21. Freedman M. Vaginal pH, estrogen and genital atrophy. Menopause Manag 17:9, 2008.
22. Castelo-Branco C, Cancelo MJ, Villero J, et al. Management of post-menopausal vaginal atrophy and atrophic vaginitis. Maturitas 52:546, 2005.
23. Archer DF. Efficacy and tolerability of local oestrogen therapy for urogenital atrophy. Menopause 17:1984, 2010.
24. Ong MW, Bashir SJ. Fractional laser resurfacing for acne scars: a review. Br J Dermatol 166:1160, 2012.
25. Peterson JD, Goldman MP. Regeneration of the aging chest: a review and our experience. Dermatol Surg 37:555, 2011.
26. Berlin AL, Hussain M, Phelps R, et al. A prospective study of fractional scanning non-sequential carbon dioxide laser resurfacing: a clinical and histopathological evaluation. Dermatol Surg 35:222, 2009.
27. Tierney EP, Hanke CW. Ablative fractional CO2 laser resurfacing for the neck: prospective study and review of the literature. J Drugs Dermatol 8:723, 2009.
28. Perino A, Calligaro A, Forlani F, et al. Vulvo-vaginal atrophy: a new treatment modality using thermo-ablative fractional CO2 laser. Maturitas 80:296, 2015.
29. Gaspar A, Addamo G, Brandi H. Vaginal fractional CO2 laser: a minimally invasive option for vaginal rejuvenation. Am J Cosmet Surg 28:156, 2011.
30. Salvatore S, Nappi RE, Zerbinati N, et al. A 12-week treatment with fractional CO2 laser for vulvovaginal atrophy: a pilot study. Climacteric 17:363, 2014.
31. Alinsod RM. Transcutaneous temperature controlled radiofrequency for atrophic vaginitis and dyspareunia. From Abstracts of the Forty-fourth AAGL Global Congress of Minimally Invasive Gynecology, Las Vegas, Nevada, Nov 2015.
32. Zerbinati N, Serati M, Origoni M, et al. Microscopic and ultrastructural modification of post-menopausal atrophic vaginal mucosa after fractional carbon dioxide laser treatment. Lasers Med Sci 30:429, 2015.
33. Millheiser LS, Pauls RN, Herbst SJ, et al. Radiofrequency treatment of vaginal laxity after vaginal delivery: nonsurgical tightening. J Sex Med 7:3088, 2010.
34. Sekiguchi Y, Utsugisawa Y, Azekosi Y, et al. Laxity of the vaginal introitus after childbirth: non-surgical outpatient procedure for vaginal tissue restoration and improving sexual satisfaction using low-energy, radiofrequency thermal therapy. J Womens Health (Larchout) 22:775, 2013.
35. Alinsod RM. Temperature controlled radiofrequency for vulvovaginal laxity. Prime Int J Aesthet Anti-Ageing Med 3:16, 2015.
36. Weiss RA, Weiss MA, Munavalli G, et al. Monopolar radio-frequency facial tightening: a retrospective analysis of efficacy and safety in our 600 treatments. J Drugs Dermatol 5:707, 2006.
37. Dover JS, Zelickson B; 14-Physician Multispecialty Consensus Panel. Results of a survey of 5,700 patient monopolar radio-frequency facial skin tightening treatments: assessment of a low-energy, multiple-pass technique leading to a clinical end point algorithm. Dermatol Surg 33:900, 2007.
38. Fitzpatrick R, Geronemus R, Goldberg D, et al. Multicenter study of noninvasive radiofrequency for periorbital tissue tightening. Lasers Surg Med 33:232, 2003.
39. Hodkinson DJ. Clinical applications of radiofrequency: nonsurgical skin tightening (thermage). Clin Plast Surg 36:261, 2009.
40. Alinsod RM. Temperature-controlled radiofrequency for vulvovaginal laxity: a pilot study. Personal communication. Thermi Health 1:1, 2015.

CHAPTER 15

O-Shot®

Charles Runels

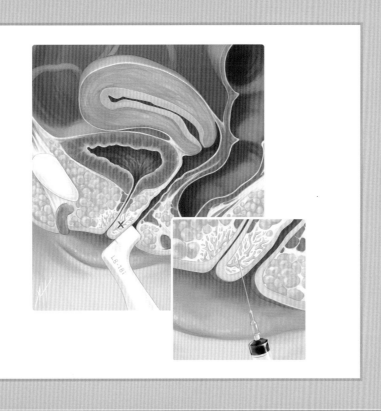

Key Points

- *The treatment of female sexual dysfunction calls for new therapies that directly affect the female genitalia.*

- *Specifically placed injections of platelet-rich plasma (PRP), the O-Shot® procedure, offer promise for female sexual dysfunction, lichen sclerosus, and urinary incontinence.*

- *Because the definition of the "G-spot" by some authors can be nebulous or functional rather than anatomic, and because anatomic descriptions may describe an area different from what we intend for the location of the injection, we propose the name "O-spot," for the most distal place between the urethra and vaginal wall, as a way of unequivocally defining one of the locations for the injection of PRP.*

- *The treatment of female sexual dysfunction has advanced so that the same systems analysis used to understand pathophysiology for other systems (such as respiration and digestion) seems warranted. Therefore the term "female orgasm system" is proposed as a useful concept.*

- *As more effective sexual therapies become available, the ethics of who can decide when "good" is "good enough" could become relevant.*

Injection of Autologous Platelet-Rich Plasma for Female Sexual Dysfunction

Approximately 40% of women have psychological distress from female sexual dysfunction, whereas only 14% of women—during their entire lifetime—will consult a physician about sex.[1] The main reason for the lack of communication about sex between women and their physicians may be that physicians avoid the conversation, thinking that solutions are few; therefore discussions are futile.[1]

As late as the 1980s, researchers advised urologists to become "primary [psycho-] therapists" to treat erectile dysfunction (ED), because "most instances of acquired impotence" were thought to be "psychogenic."[2] The FDA approved more than 20 drugs to help men with ED, after research demonstrated that most cases of ED arose not from psychological causes, but instead from neurovascular and endocrine disorders.[3] Or, did new therapies addressing neurovascular causes of ED facilitate better understanding of the cause?[3]

Conversely, for women, the class A drug therapies for FSD currently include only "short-term" testosterone and the one drug approved by the FDA for FSD, flibanserin.[1,4]

No FDA-approved drug for FSD directly targets the female genitalia.[1] Flibanserin affects women by altering serotonin and dopamine levels with no direct effect on the genitalia, placing the drug in the same class as an antidepressant. Furthermore, no form of testosterone for women is currently approved by the FDA. Because the clitoris is analogous to the penis in anatomy and physiology,[5] and because men have sexual dysfunction secondary to penile pathology (for example, from autoimmune disease, decreased circulation, or loss of sensation), then future treatments for women that might directly address pathology of the genitalia are plausible.

Because phosphodiesterase inhibitors (PDEIs) help men with sexual dysfunction, the same strategy could seem plausible for women. However, on closer examination of the benefits PDEIs provide men, the crossover seems less promising with this class of drugs. Although PDEIs improve firmness of the penis by altering hemodynamics, they do little to correct the pathophysiology that necessitates their use.[6] This shortfall prompted a call for therapies that correct the primary causes of erectile dysfunction.[6] Moreover, the simple achievement of the mechanical state of rigid cavernosi through increased tumescence would directly solve a problem for men (the need for a penis rigid enough for sexual intercourse) but at best would only secondarily correct female sexual dysfunction, because a rigid clitoris solves no particular female sexual dysfunction. Nor do rigid corpus cavernosi primarily solve the male sexual dysfunctions that are analogous to those found in women (decreased libido, decreased sensation, pain with intercourse, or decreased ability to orgasm). Nevertheless, even though erect corpi would not directly solve any particular female sexual dysfunction, the idea showed promise in some studies, although they showed "significant increases in adverse events compared to placebo."[7] Furthermore, even though the treatment of FSD often requires the use of psychological and endocrine modalities, the extension of that idea—that therapies directly affecting the female genitalia offer little benefit—seems limiting and unlikely. For example, a woman may not enjoy benefit from a drug directed toward the brain if she has scarring from an episiotomy or from lichen sclerosus, pain from pelvic floor tenderness, or anorgasmia from diabetes with neurovascular compromise of the clitoris. Therefore more class A therapies (drugs and procedures) for women directed to the pathology of the female genitalia are needed.

Orgasms: More and More Intense

A subset of women with FSD (1 of 20) has female orgasmic disorder: either difficulty achieving or complete inability to experience orgasm.[1] Successful treatment of orgasmic disorder not only improves a woman's sexual pleasure but also can improve her emotional bonding, mental health, and relationships.[4]

Although testosterone therapy can facilitate female orgasm (partly by maintaining the integrity of the vaginal nerve fiber network and muscularis volume while enhancing genital blood flow and mucification), women who cannot use testosterone or who already have normal levels of the hormone have only psychotherapy as their primary class A treatment.[1,8-10] All drug strategies, including flibanserin and testosterone, are off label—not approved by the FDA—for the treatment of female orgasmic disorder.

Medications provide few options for improving female orgasm; thus the available procedures are considered. Hyaluronic acid (HA) gel and collagen have been injected into the G-spot to enhance orgasm in women by facilitating increased pressure on the G-spot during sexual intercourse; but these therapies were not designed to treat sexual dysfunction (only to improve normal function) and are not known to propagate the repair of tissue.[11,12] Moreover, because erosion, urinary obstruction, and pulmonary embolus are risks in women undergoing HA enhancement of the G-spot, the American College of Obstetrics and Gynecology published a position paper to discourage physicians from providing the procedure.[13-15]

Similarly, the FDA approved calcium hydroxyapatite crystals (Coaptite) for injection near the urethra for the relief of urinary stress incontinence, but such use risks foreign body granuloma formation resulting in erosion or obstruction, requiring surgical correction in about 1 in 40 women.[16,17] Although still FDA approved for urinary incontinence, Coaptite is neither indicated nor suggested as a treatment for FSD.[18]

The idea of injecting material near the urethra to improve sexual function or to stop urinary incontinence has been discussed for more than a decade. The challenge has been to find a material that provides therapeutic benefits without unacceptable adverse effects.[19]

A new and exciting treatment involves the use of PRP to enhance female sexual function.[20] In contrast to the above-mentioned synthetic materials, PRP has been shown to have no serious adverse effects and to be effective in multiple studies for the treatment of soft tissue wounds and joint injury and for orthopedic and dental surgery and a variety of cosmetic procedures.[21-23] Pluripotent stem cells exposed to PRP activate and develop into new tissue—nerve, collagen, and blood vessels.[24-26] Moreover, the medical literature contains many articles demonstrating the safety of PRP, with no reports of granuloma formation, infection, or any other serious adverse effects when the laboratory equipment used has been approved by the FDA for the preparation of PRP for use in the body.[26,27] PRP is even used to treat scarring and to restore atrophied tissue; the possibility of causing scarring from PRP is theoretically impossible.[28,29] Because PRP is aqueous, it flows easily through a small-bore needle (for patient comfort with only local anesthesia) and is evenly distributed (which prevents the need for the meticulous positioning of the needle required for injecting an HA gel or a calcium hydroxyapatite crystal slurry).[30]

A pilot study was conducted to determine the effects of specifically placed, localized injections of PRP for the treatment of FSD, the O-Shot procedure.[30] As described in this chapter, the in-office procedure takes about 15 minutes.

First, a topical anesthetic is applied to the introitus and clitoris. Whole blood is then drawn from the arm and processed at the bedside to extract PRP using a kit approved by the FDA for PRP preparation for injection back into the body.[31,32] With the woman in a lithotomy position, 4 ml of her PRP is activated with 0.2 ml of 10% calcium chloride and injected into the O-spot—the space between the urethra and the vaginal wall, most distally, in the area of the periurethral glands (Figs. 15-1 and 15-2). One milliliter of activated PRP is injected into the clitoral corpus cavernosum, near the glans clitoris.

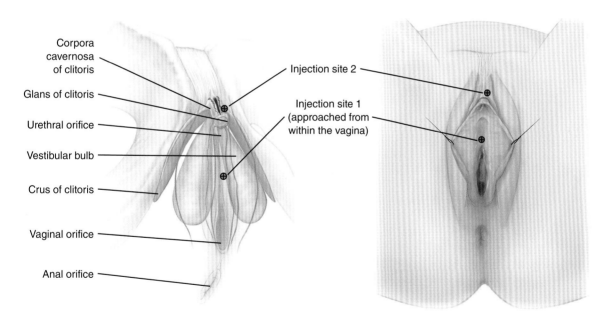

Fig. 15-1   Injection of 4 ml of PRP at the O-spot *(injection site 1)*. Fluid fills the tissue between the urethra and the vagina. Injection of 1 ml into the body of the corpus cavernosum *(injection site 2)*. Ultrasonography performed during the procedures demonstrated fluid passing into all parts of the clitoris and completely bathing the Skene glands. Immediate changes in the ureterovesicular angle were observed.

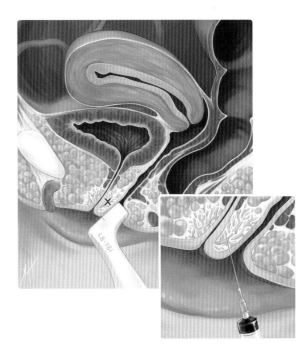

Fig. 15-2 Endovaginal placement of the hockey-stick–shaped 18 MHz ultrasound probe shows a urethral curvilinear echo, with circumferential periurethral smooth muscle and areolar tissue between the urethra and vagina in the area of the O-spot *(X)*. Ultrasound images obtained during and after the O-Shot procedure demonstrated hyrodissection of the area by the injected PRP.

In a study of the O-Shot procedure, after 12 to 16 weeks and only one injection, two standardized tests were used to measure the effects of the procedure: the Female Sexual Distress Scale-Revised (FSDS-R) and the Female Sexual Function Index (FSFI).[32,33] The FSDS-R questionnaire measures sexually related distress (a score of 11 or more indicates distress).[33] The FSFI questionnaire measures arousal, desire, pain, orgasm, satisfaction, and lubrication.[34]

In the same study, 7 of 10 (70%) women progressed from *distressed* to *not distressed,* with reported scores that decreased an average of 10 points on the FSDS-R, from a mean of 17 to 7 ($p = 0.04$).[30] Responses on the FSFI questionnaire were measured. Eight of 10 women showed a statistically significant improvement in the domains of desire, arousal, lubrication, and orgasm, with a mean improvement of 5.5. Satisfaction, though trending toward statistical significance, showed less improvement partly because the woman's libido increased in some cases beyond the level of her partner's desire, resulting in frustration and therefore less improvement in satisfaction despite improvement in other domains.

The explanation for the demonstrated marked improvements may be multifactorial, as indicated by other recent supportive studies. One such study showed that women who easily achieve orgasm are more likely than women with orgasmic disorder to demonstrate on MRI studies of the clitoris both a larger clitoris and a clitoris positioned closer to the vaginal wall.[35] Because PRP has been shown to propagate new, healthy tissue of multiple cell types, the effect of PRP on the clitoral corpus cavernosum could be to enhance sensation by improving the health and function of tissue allowing communication of the clitoris with the vaginal wall. The relation of the functional anatomy to the production of orgasm is widely disputed,[5] and variations of the proposed technique could prove more effective and help to further define the mechanisms involved. Perhaps larger amounts injected into the clitoris would be beneficial. In some cases of dyspareunia, trigger point injections of the pelvic floor were helpful, as were multiple injections of episiotomy scars in combination with the described technique.

Improved sexual function in women is correlated with increased blood flow through the clitoris.[36] Because the PRP-derived growth factor known as *vascular endothelial growth factor* (or VEGF) is known to cause neovascularization, part of the effect of the O-Shot procedure may be secondary to improved blood flow through both the clitoris and the periurethral space.[37]

Injecting the O-spot may cause proliferation and activation of the periurethral glands, accounting for the onset of ejaculation with the associated increase in orgasm seen in some women after the procedure.[30]

Parenthetically, no stem cells per se are used in this method, only PRP. Some studies combine PRP with stem cells without distinguishing which of the two may be more helpful.[38] Although stem cell therapies hold promise, mesenchymal stem cells are classified as a drug by the FDA and require an extra level of expense, time, and vigilance. Alternatively, pluripotent stem cells lie dormant in the native tissue and are responsible for normal wound healing with no stem cell transfer needed, because PRP activates local mesenchymal stem cells and pericytes while releasing cytokines, which recruit other regenerative cells to the area.[37]

The O-Shot procedure has other possible indications. In a recent study using only PRP (without mesenchymal stem cells), this same methodology decreased inflammation (determined by two blinded dermatopathologists) and provided a statistical improvement of the symptoms of women with lichen sclerosus.[39] The advantage of O-Shot methodology over topical steroids for lichen sclerosus could include resolution of scarring secondary to lichen sclerosus.[28,29] PRP may enhance the immune system; thus using it to treat lichen sclerosus might lower the risk of neoplasia that occurs when it is treated with steroids in the presence of human papilloma virus infection.[40,41]

The nerves for both micturition and sexual response may be improved by PRP if the effects of PRP in the vagina mirror those seen in other tissues in previous studies.[42] Therefore this procedure holds promise for the treatment of both stress and urge urinary incontinence.

The O-Shot procedure also may improve outcome when combined with radiofrequency or laser therapy applied to the vaginal wall in the same way that PRP improves outcome and hastens recovery after laser therapy of the face, as shown in cosmetic studies.[43]

Possible contraindications to the procedure, in general, include conditions that interfere with wound healing and could negatively affect the outcome: smoking, high-dose corticosteroids, and significant thrombocytopenia. Pregnancy and psychological disorders are relative contraindications. Chronic antiplatelet therapy has been considered a relative contraindication, but studies have suggested positive outcomes even in the presence of these therapies.[44] The O-Shot procedure has no absolute contraindications, because it uses autologous plasma; there are no reports of serious side effects from PRP alone in more than 8000 papers published. Greater volumes than suggested injected into the O-spot by one provider resulted in one case of overflow obstruction that resolved without sequelae. Bruising, hypersexuality, and mild dysuria have been the only side effects observed thus far.

The Female Orgasm System: The Time Has Come

A *system* consists of interacting elements forming a complex whole with regard to its purposes.[45] When considering a particular therapy for sexual dysfunction, whether it be drugs that target the brain, psychotherapy, hormonal therapies, or local therapies, it may be helpful to apply systems analysis.[46] If the respiratory system, circulatory system, and renal system can be better understood and researched and patients better treated using systems analysis, then patients might benefit from a similar thought process applied to female orgasm and arousal.[47,48]

The reproductive system shares components with the orgasm system, so why the redundancy? Arousal and orgasm bring pleasure and bonding but do not always lead to pregnancy (the purpose of the reproductive system) and pregnancy may occur without arousal or orgasm (the purpose of the orgasm system). Thus we propose that defining the components needed for sexual pleasure and orgasm and mapping the interactions of these components using systems analysis could help to overcome the shortfalls of thinking compartmentally about these systems. Even when analyzing normal function, considering arousal and orgasm as the result of an operating system encourages more effective strategies for optimizing outcome.

Not long ago, the clitoris was not illustrated in *Gray's Anatomy,* and a detailed analysis of hormones was not available; the function of the Skene glands was not known, and the vagina was arguably thought of as only a birth canal and a receptacle for a penis; the high incidence of FSD was unrecognized, and the idea of an orgasm system was not needed. But with deeper understanding comes the need for a more thoughtful organization of ideas. For example, using systems analysis prevents the narrow focus that results in attempts to relieve dyspareunia with psychotherapy (when an alternative treatment may have resolved pain) or to increase libido with only testosterone (for abused women and those in a strained relationship). Systems analysis encourages patients and practitioners from multiple disciplines to consider the entire spectrum of available therapies and to more strategically cooperate in finding health and healing.

The female orgasm system comprises at least the following components: (1) endocrine, (2) neurogenic, (3) vascular, (4) anatomic/mechanical, (5) pharmacologic, (6) emotional, and (7) relational.[49]

The female orgasm system needs more thought by researchers to define the components, how the components interact, and how those interactions may be optimized. For example, systems analysis applied to recent anatomic studies spawned the idea of the clitourethro-vaginal complex as a more elegant descriptor of the anatomy responsible for arousal than the traditional G-spot.[50]

As another example of systems thinking, aerobic exercise by women taking antidepressants alters dopamine and serotonin, leading to improved sexual function for about 1 hour.[51] Trained athletes with high aerobic capacity, compared with matched sedentary women, demonstrated increased clitoral blood flow associated with improved sexual function and reported higher scores on the FSFI in the domains of arousal and orgasm.[52] Mapping the multiple changes in the female orgasm system seen with elite physical training is useful for understanding how systems analysis facilitates both the planning of specific therapies and future research. It also helps to understand how the O-Shot procedure could fit into this systems-structured treatment plan.

Systems analysis allows physicians to optimize a system that is functioning "normally." Thus continued research presents an important question: Is it ethical to help a woman with normal sexual function to achieve better function? Currently, it is considered unethical for physicians to give normally functioning patients hormones for muscle enhancement. Is there a level of *normal* that makes it unethical to help women discover more sexual pleasure? Specifically, is it ethical for physicians to prescribe to enhance sexual pleasure and not only to treat disease? If not, then where is the line that distinguishes disease from normal, and who should draw it: the physician or each woman?

Considered from a systems perspective, the O-Shot is not a magic cure-all but instead only a way of potentially promoting healthier, more functional vaginal tissue—nothing more, nothing less. Every other proven tool still applies.

As more therapies evolve, systems analysis and ethical issues will become more important to the treatment of FSD.

References

1. American College of Obstetricians and Gynecologists Committee on Practice Bulletins-Gynecology. ACOG Practice Bulletin No. 119: Female sexual dysfunction. Obstet Gynecol 117:996, 2011.
2. Finkle AL. Sexual impotency: current knowledge and treatment I. Urology/sexuality clinic. Urology 16:449, 1980.
3. Basu A, Ryder RE. New treatment options for erectile dysfunction in patients with diabetes mellitus. Drugs 64:2667, 2004.

CHAPTER 16

Transcutaneous Temperature-Controlled Radiofrequency for Vulvovaginal Rejuvenation

Red Alinsod

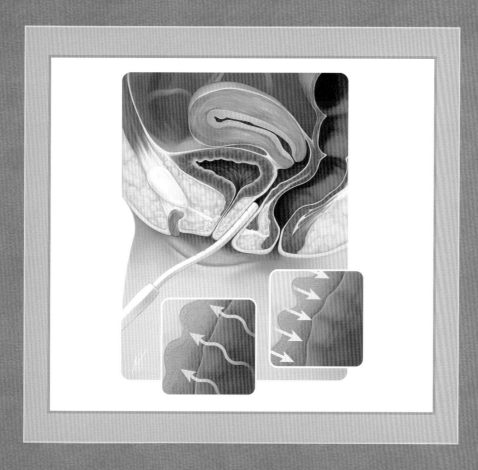

Key Points

- *Temperature-controlled radiofrequency (RF) tightens vulvovaginal tissues immediately and over a period of several months and is effective for nonsurgical vulvar and vaginal tightening.*

- *Temperature-controlled RF encourages new collagen formation and neoangiogenesis, resulting in improved skin tone and sensitivity.*

- *Tightening of vaginal tissues reduces vaginal laxity, stress incontinence, overactive bladder, and mild to moderate cystocele and rectocele.*

- *Temperature-controlled RF results in improved vulvovaginal blood flow that normalizes vaginal moisture and improves overall sensitivity of the clitoral, vulvar, and vaginal tissues.*

- *Orgasmic dysfunction may be aided by temperature-controlled RF treatments.*

Between childbirth—often multiple childbirths—and waning estrogen levels from menopause, the vagina undergoes numerous changes that lead to a well-defined suite of conditions that begins with vulvovaginal laxity with reduced elasticity and includes atrophic vaginitis (leading to chronic irritation and discomfort), stress urinary incontinence, and different manifestations of sexual dysfunction. Any or all of these may be present, and the age of onset may vary. Addressing these conditions is problematic because of two factors. First, women have traditionally had difficulty discussing these issues with their primary care physician or gynecologist. Until recently, social mores were responsible for a dim view of frank discussions about the vagina, and the societal attitude toward these

---

I first used radiofrequency for precision labial surgery in 2005. The concept for intravaginal and vulvar use of radiofrequency became a reality in 2009-2010 when I performed the first radiofrequency treatments on the vulvovaginal area for aesthetic benefits of tissue shrinkage. In 2013 I started development of ThermiVa (Thermi), a specific device intended for use on both the vulva and the deep vagina for the purpose of dermal skin tightening and vaginal tightening. Clinical research showed that the vaginal and anal mucosal treatments and tissue tightening also aided in relief of stress incontinence, overactive bladder, mild to moderate cystocele and rectocele, orgasmic dysfunction, and fecal incontinence. I continue to consult with Thermi and perform clinical studies on the effects of temperature-controlled RF in vulvovaginal tissues. ThermiVa is FDA approved for dermatologic conditions and surgical nerve ablation in the United States. Examples of dermatologic conditions are loose skin, dry skin, and insensitive skin. ThermiVa does not currently have specific FDA approval for vaginal or anal tightening, vulvovaginal atrophy, stress incontinence, overactive bladder, pelvic prolapse, fecal incontinence, and organic dysfunction. I receive royalties from the sale of ThermiVa generators and wands.

conditions was one of resignation. Second, physicians' armamentarium has been anything but comprehensive, limited to hormone therapy, Kegel exercises to strengthen the pelvic floor, the use of creams or lubricants, and more invasive surgical options.

Energy-based modalities have been applied to this tissue in the same fashion as in aesthetic medicine, with the purpose of causing collagen denaturation and contracture, stimulating neocollagenesis and feminine restoration through the healing cascade from the heating of tissue. This thermal effect induces the production of fibroblasts and stimulates neocollagenesis. Intuitively, the ability to deliver more energy will cause a more profound effect, to a point. Directed energy does not cause the sensation of pain in the vaginal wall as readily as it does in facial skin, making energy-based therapies more tolerable at higher energies, and suggesting that the vagina may be an ideal anatomic region for energy-based resurfacing of tissue. Regardless of which term is used—rejuvenation, resurfacing, tightening, or treatment of laxity—the basic aims and methods are similar.

Tissue contraction using RF energy is an established modality in aesthetic medicine.[1,2] Heat is generated in proximity to the electrode through impedance as RF energy travels through tissue, which can be calculated using an equation accounting for local electrical conductivity and the level of current generated near the electrode (RF emitter).[3] This specific pattern of thermogenesis is thus predictable and can be controlled by modulating power to the electrode itself. Therapeutically relevant heating of tissue has been shown to lie within a recognized temperature range (40° to 45° C) to optimally stimulate neocollagenesis and neoelastinogenesis while minimizing collateral damage to skin and nearby tissue structures; RF energy must therefore be controlled in relation to tissue temperature during therapy to maximize energy delivery, yet prevent overtreatment. Unlike other proven energy-based methods, RF is completely noninvasive; thus skin barrier function is preserved, minimizing healing time and patient risk. Because RF does not use light energy, skin pigmentation is not a factor in treatment. RF energy is especially suited for naturally moist and well-hydrated tissue such as that of the vaginal wall and vulva.[4]

Transcutaneous temperature-controlled RF (TTCRF) therapy, brand name ThermiVa, employs a monopolar RF electrode and return pad (to complete the circuit), between which electric current is passed.[3,4] Power to the RF emitter is automatically modulated by thermistors and thermocouples integrated into the treatment device to monitor local tissue temperature in real time. Thus temperature targets may be safely achieved rapidly and maintained for a duration sufficient for therapeutic tissue response. Proper management of tissue temperature has a positive impact on patient comfort during treatment; treatment is very comfortable and no anesthesia is necessary.

For vaginal applications,[4] TTCRF technology is contained within a treatment probe approximately 20 cm long and 1.5 cm wide (about the width of an adult finger) with a shallow S curve toward the center, similar to that of a Hegar dilator (Fig. 16-1). The slim treatment probe has the advantage of reducing potential trauma from insertion resulting from dryness, sensitivity, and atrophy of vaginal wall tissue. The RF emitter (about the size of a postage stamp) is located on one side of the probe tip.

During treatment the patient rests comfortably in the dorsal lithotomy position. The probe is inserted into the vagina, with the RF emitter facing the tissue in the treatment zone; externally, the RF emitter is applied directly to vulvar structures. (The vulva can be shaved.) Potential treatment zones include the dorsal, ventral, left, and right vaginal wall and vulvar structures. The probe is then passed over each treatment zone continuously until the target temperature has been achieved and maintained for 3 to 5 minutes or longer (based on the patient's tolerance).

Treatment is safe enough to be regionally concentrated, for example, along pubocervical fascia for treating stress urinary incontinence or on and around the G-spot, clitoral hood, and clitoral area for treating orgasmic dysfunction. No preparatory or posttreatment protocol is required; therefore patients may return to normal activity immediately after treatment and need not abstain from sex.

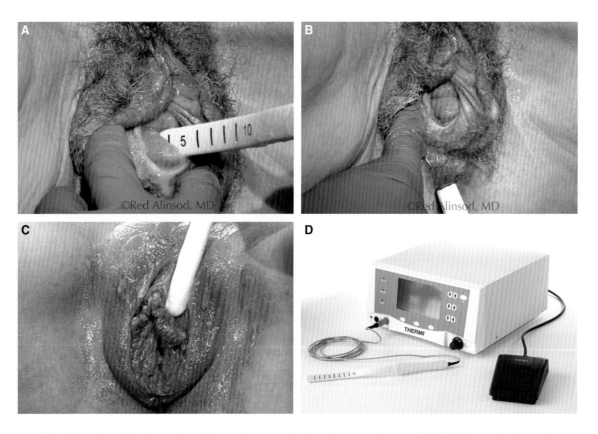

Fig. 16-1   A and **B,** Examples of internal transvaginal and transanal use of TTCRF. The probe is small in relation to the vaginal anatomy, allowing comfortable treatment in even the most extreme cases of vaginal wall atrophy and atrophic vaginitis. Transanal treatments for rectocele, fecal incontinence, internal hemorrhoids, and anal laxity are currently being studied in the United States and abroad. **C,** Example of vulvar and clitoral hood treatment. **D,** The ThermiVa Box is compact, lightweight, and easily portable.

A typical course of treatment includes up to three sessions, with 4 to 6 weeks between treatments to allow time for tissue remodeling. Yearly maintenance treatments may be beneficial. A complete course of vulvovaginal TTCRF treatment typically results in an aesthetic enhancement of the vulva, tightening of the vaginal mucosa, and improvement in tissue elasticity. Improvement in tissue quality and increased local blood flow lead to improvement in production of lubrication and transudate. Personal communication of a pending publication by Drs. Gustavo Leibashoff and Pablo Gonzales, in Columbia, has confirmed histologic evidence that TTCRF treatments increase vulvar and vaginal collagen production and neoangiogenesis, as well as thickening of vulvar and vaginal surfaces, and improves the maturation index. Their study has shown that TTCRF seems to be a promising alternative for the treatment of mild to moderate stress urinary incontinence and other symptoms related to genitourinary syndrome of menopause. In collaboration with John Miklos and Robert Moore, their work has been published.[5]

Potential ancillary effects may include improvements in related conditions. Early investigation has shown improvement of up to 25% and greater than 33% for overactive bladder with and without incontinence, respectively[6]; reduction in average time to orgasm of up to 50% for patients with orgasmic dysfunction and orgasm restoration for anorgasmic patients[7]; average improvement of 2.5 points on the Sexual Satisfaction Scale and 5 points on the Vaginal Laxity Questionnaire, and reduction or elimination of the need for lubricants for patients with atrophic vulvovaginitis and dyspareunia[8]; resolution of severe vaginal stenosis[8]; and improvement in mild to moderate stress urinary incontinence.[4,8,9] In some cases, reduction or elimination of vaginal estrogen therapy has been noted after TTCRF.[4,8] Anecdotal evidence of successful treatment of cystocele (transvaginally) and rectocele (using transvaginal and transanal TTCRF) has also been reported (Fig. 16-2). TTCRF holds much promise as a safe and effective noninvasive, nonsurgical, nonpharmacologic, nonsteroidal modality with numerous potential therapeutic applications.

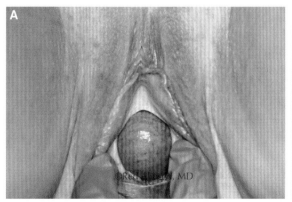 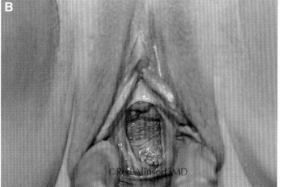

Fig. 16-2 This 56-year-old menopausal woman had pelvic pressure and a vaginal bulge, as well as an overactive bladder and stress incontinence. **A,** The cystocele is shown on maximum Valsalva maneuver before treatment. **B,** One treatment with TTCRF reduced the bulge, overactive bladder, and incontinence, preventing the need for surgical repair and anticholinergic medication.

Results

Two years of ongoing clinical studies at our center and multiple centers worldwide have shown exceptionally safe treatments with temperature-controlled RF. In its first year of release in the United States and worldwide, more than 10,000 women have been safely treated with ThermiVa. No blisters or burns or serious adverse events have been reported or seen with several thousand treatments. ThermiVa treatments are well tolerated and satisfaction rates high. Shrinkage of labia majora tissue is often dramatic and quite evident, although the labia minora shrinkage is more modest at approximately 20%. The vaginal tightening effects can be significant for both the patient and partner, with improved vaginal moisture seen without the use of hormones or lubricants. Dyspareunia can be reduced and eliminated. ThermiVa is becoming a widely and rapidly accepted treatment for mild to moderate stress incontinence, overactive bladder without incontinence, mild

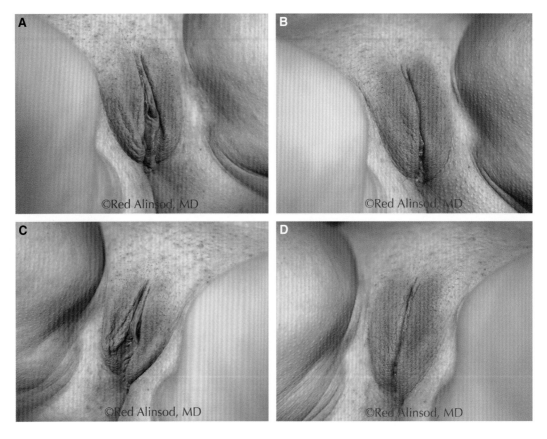

Fig. 16-3   A and **C,** This 57-year-old multiparous woman is shown before three TTCRF treatments for vulvovaginal atrophy and laxity, stress urinary incontinence, and orgasmic dysfunction. **B** and **D,** Post-operatively, resolution of her symptoms is dramatic.

to moderate cystocele and rectocele, and orgasmic dysfunction; more recently, it has been used as a novel treatment for certain types of fecal incontinence and anal laxity. ThermiVa does not have specific FDA clearance for these conditions as they continue to be studied, but it is approved for dermatologic conditions and surgical nerve ablation, as mentioned earlier. ThermiVa does not appear to be as effective for severe stress incontinence, intrinsic sphincter deficiency, detrusor overactivity/instability, and overactive bladder with incontinence. Current studies are evaluating the efficacy of ThermiVa use in conjunction with platelet-rich plasma. Results of various treatments are shown in Figs. 16-3 through 16-6.

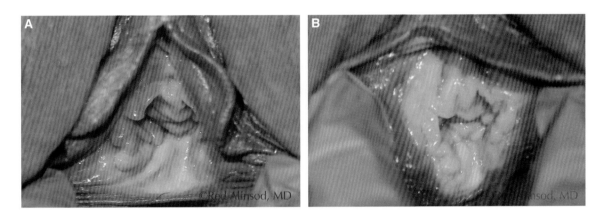

Fig. 16-4   A, This multiparous perimenopausal woman in her mid-40s had vaginal dryness and laxity. **B,** After two treatments with TTCRF, her tissue is notably tighter and more plump, with visible improvement in transudate.

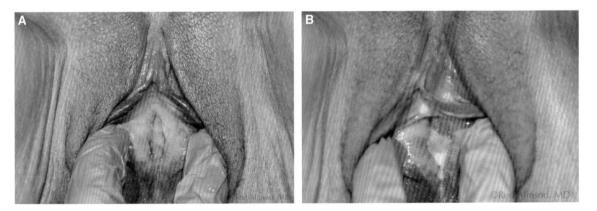

Fig. 16-5   A, This menopausal woman in her mid-60s had vaginal dryness and dyspareunia. **B,** After two treatments with TTCRF, her tissue is notably more moist and more elastic.

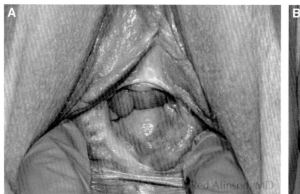 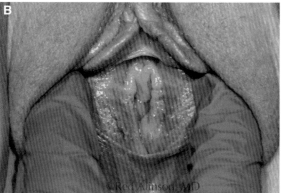

Fig. 16-6 **A,** This 62-year-old menopausal woman presented with vaginal laxity, stress incontinence, and a rectocele. **B,** After three treatments with TTCRF, her tissue shrinkage is dramatic, and her symptoms have resolved without the need for surgery.

References

1. Mulholland RS. Radio frequency energy for non-invasive and minimally invasive skin tightening. Clin Plast Surg 38:437, 2011.
2. Dunbar SW, Goldberg DJ. Radiofrequency in dermatology: an update. J Drugs Dermatol 14:1229, 2015.
3. Key DJ. Integration of thermal imaging with subsurface radiofrequency thermistor heating for the purpose of skin tightening and contour improvement: a retrospective review of clinical efficacy. J Drugs Dermatol 13:1485, 2014.
4. Alinsod RM. Temperature controlled radiofrequency for vulvovaginal laxity. Prime: Int J Aesthet Anti-Ageing Med 3:16, 2015.
5. Leibaschoff G, Izasa PG, Cardona JL, et al. Transcutaneous temperature controlled radiofrequency (TTCRF) for the treatment of menopausal vaginal/genitourinary symptoms. Surg Technol Int 2016 Sept 10. [Epub ahead of print]
6. Alinsod RM. Transcutaneous temperature controlled radiofrequency for overactive bladder. Abstract accepted for presentation at the Forty-first Annual Meeting of the International Urogynecological Association, Cape Town, South Africa, Aug 2016.
7. Alinsod RM. Transcutaneous temperature controlled radiofrequency for orgasmic dysfunction. Lasers Surg Med 48:641, 2016.
8. Alinsod RM. Transcutaneous temperature controlled radiofrequency for atrophic vaginitis and dyspareunia. J Minim Invasive Gynecol 22:S226, 2015.
9. Magon N, Alinsod RM. ThermiVa: the revolutionary technology for vulvovaginal rejuvenation and noninvasive management of female SUI. J Obstet Gynaecol India 66:300, 2016.

CHAPTER 17

Fractional Erbium Laser for Vaginal Rejuvenation

Evgenii Leshunov

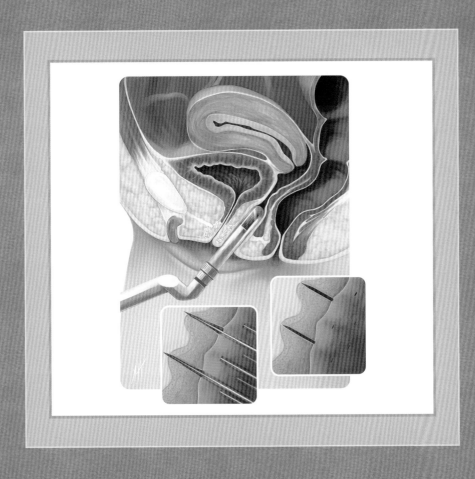

Key Points

- *Er:YAG 2940 nm is one of the most popular systems for laser vaginal rejuvenation in the world.*

- *This technology has been used to treat the syndrome of vaginal relaxation, stress urinary incontinence, and vaginal atrophy.*

- *Fractional vaginal rejuvenation is a simple outpatient procedure that requires no anesthesia.*

- *The rehabilitation period after vaginal rejuvenation with the use of an erbium laser is 72 hours.*

Fractional Er:YAG systems with a dedicated gynecological delivery system recently became commercially available.

Er:YAG systems offer a nonsurgical approach for vaginal tightening. Erbium laser technology is used for treating vaginal laxity, stress urinary incontinence, pelvic organ prolapsed, and vaginal atrophy. The first trials for erbium tightening of the vaginal canal began in 2008 and 2009.[1]

From 2010 to 2014 several clinical studies involving all four indications were conducted to prove the efficacy and safety of this novel technology. The infrared erbium (Er:YAG) laser has an emission wavelength of 2.94 μ and operates in pulse mode. The main mechanism of action of the laser technology is selective stimulation of the submucosal (lamina propria) collagen synthesis and thermal stimulation of mucosal tissue. The instantaneous reaction of contraction in the collagen fibers and acceleration of neocollagenesis lead to the contraction of tissues and an increase in their elasticity.

The choice of the Er:YAG with its 2940 nm wavelength for this gynecological probe-based system was predicated on the absorption peak of water at that wavelength. Human tissues are a good target for this wavelength because of their very high percentage of water, especially in the vaginal area where mucous membranes are present and in the lamina propria (submucosal area). Because of the extremely high absorption in water, the

Dr. Leshunov consults and presents at congresses for Asclepion Laser Technologies.

incident photon energy is almost totally quenched in the first micrometers of tissue, producing at appropriate parameters a very controlled column of thermal stimulation with an extremely narrow band of secondary coagulation, known as *residual thermal damage.*[2]

Collagen is an important component of pelvic floor supportive structures—it makes up more than 80% of the protein content of the endopelvic fascia. Collagen provides tensile strength and integrity, and elastin is responsible for the elasticity and resilience of the connective tissue of the pelvic floor. The extracellular matrix of the vaginal wall consists of collagen type I, III, and V. The ratio of collagen type I/type III determines the mechanical properties of the vaginal wall. A change in the ratio toward collagen type III, which is most frequently observed in vaginal prolapse and stress incontinence, can significantly reduce the elasticity of the vaginal wall.

Collagen type V is an important component of basement membranes. Changes in the condition of this collagen are very rare. Elastin helps to provide support to the pelvic floor. With age, decreased elastin in the extracellular matrix causes a loss of submucosal supporting function of the vaginal wall.[3]

Pelvic tissue from women with stress urinary incontinence and pelvic organ prolapse shows a genetic predisposition to abnormal extracellular matrix remodeling, which is modulated by reproductive hormones, trauma, mechanical stress load, and aging. This progressive remodeling contributes to stress urinary incontinence and pelvic organ prolapse by altering normal tissue architecture and mechanical properties. Laser-mediated mechanical and heat pulsing of the endopelvic fascia and pelvic floor tissue could be an effective nonsurgical method for treating female urinary incontinence and other disorders resulting from diminished pelvic floor support.

Collagen that undergoes appropriate mechanical (ablative) and/or thermal microdamage is regenerated, resulting in more elasticity, tightening in the sudden contraction of its fibers, and contraction and shrinking of the irradiated bulk tissue.[4] The result is a better response by muscular tissue in the pelvic floor.

Dr. Rodolfo Milani conducted a pilot study at the University of Milano-Bicocca, San Gerardo Hospital in Monza, Italy, to evaluate the safety and efficacy of a novel treatment protocol for vaginal rejuvenation using Er:YAG. Forty-seven patients received treatment for vaginal atrophy between December 2015 and April 2016. The average patient age was 55 years. Every 2 weeks, patients underwent a vaginal atrophy assessment (speculum examination and vaginal pH) and completed questionnaires on atrophy symptoms and quality of life (Utian Quality of Life [UQOL] Scale).[5]

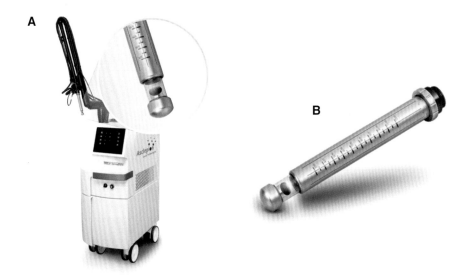

Fig. 17-1   A, MCL31 Dermablate (Er:YAG 2940 nm). **B,** Juliet vaginal probe.

At baseline and after 6 weeks, a Pap smear with a maturation index was performed and a vaginal biopsy sample cultured. The laser system used was the MCL31™ Er:YAG (Asclepion Laser Technologies), delivering a wavelength of 2940 nm (Fig. 17-1). When fitted with the dedicated vaginal probe (Juliet™ Asclepion Laser Technologies), the laser can be operated in the multiple micropulse mode (pulse width of 300 μs, selectable number of pulses in burst) and in the long-pulsed thermal mode (1000 μs, single pulse). The protocol called for one treatment session.

Punch biopsies were performed at baseline and at day 7 after treatment, formalin fixed, and routinely prepared for light microscopy with hematoxylin and eosin staining and two-photon microscopy.

All subjects completed the treatment and the 3-month assessment. All patients were aware of a heating sensation in the vagina during treatment. None reported major or lasting adverse effects after treatment.

Results

All women had a significant reduction in vaginal pH from 6.5 to 7 ($\pm$ 0.3) to 4.5 ($\pm$ 0.3). pH is one of the most important and sensitive means of evaluating the functional state of vaginal mucosa. A pH change toward alkalinity disrupts the vaginal flora and reduces the mucosal barrier function. The use of laser light changes the trophic properties of tissue. It increases blood circulation lubrication, and the level of glycosaminoglycans, promoting considerable reduction of pH and restoration of normal vaginal biocenosis.

All patients reported a subjective improvement in all symptoms of vaginal atrophy.

The vaginal maturation index (VMI) improved: Parabasal cells were 100% at entry and 33% after 6 weeks of treatment, intermediate cells changed from 0% to 40%, and superficial cells changed from 0% to 27%. The VMI is a ratio obtained by performing a random cell count of the three major cell types shed from the vaginal squamous epithelium: parabasal, intermediate, and superficial. It is reported as relative percentages of these cells and written as a ratio (parabasal %:intermediate %:superficial %).

The VMI is thought to show the effect of estrogen on the vaginal mucosa (not the cervix). Parabasal cells are not affected by estrogen and progesterone, because they are immature cells; intermediate cells are somewhat mature, having been affected by progesterone; and superficial cells are the most mature, having been affected by estrogen. A large percentage of parabasal cells can indicate a lack of estrogen affecting the tissues. A large percentage of superficial cells indicates that a lot of estrogenic stimulation has occurred. Intermediate cells have no value here.

VMI numbers are interpreted as follows: 49 or less indicates not very much, or zero, estrogenic effect; 50 to 64 indicates a moderate estrogenic effect; and 65 to 100 indicates a dominant, fertile (premenopausal), estrogenic environment.

Because we can see improvement in the trophism of the mucosa and submucosa with the use of Er:YAG, we decided to evaluate the changes of this index before and after treatment. We noted a significant improvement in the index, which returned to premenopausal levels after two laser treatment procedures.

Patients reported a significant improvement in their UQOL score, including the sexual domain of the scale.[5]

The histologic findings in general showed evidence of a thicker and more cellular epithelium and a more compact lamina propria with a denser arrangement of connective tissue, as shown in Figs. 17-2 and 17-3.

The results of the histologic analysis suggested tightening and firming of the vaginal wall.

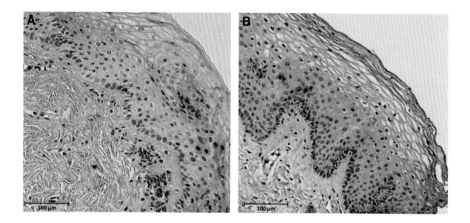

Fig. 17-2   Hematoxylin and eosin–stained specimens of the vaginal wall. **A,** Baseline sample. **B,** Seven days after treatment, mucosal architecture is improved in the epithelium and the lamina propria.

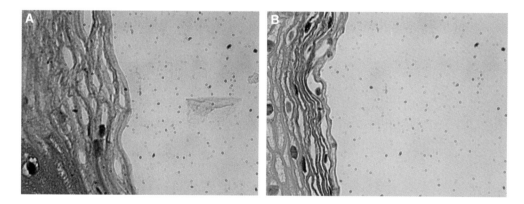

Fig. 17-3   Photon microscopy images of the vaginal wall. **A,** At baseline, the epithelium was split, with few and pyknotic nuclei. **B,** Seven days after treatment, the epithelium is multilayered and well organized with nuclei present.

Conclusion

The preliminary results of our study confirm that a minimally invasive, fractional laser treatment with short- and long-pulse Er:YAG is an effective, safe, and comfortable treatment option for vaginal rejuvenation in patients with vaginal atrophy.

All patients have subjective improvement in their sex life because of improved vaginal lubrication, more sensation during intercourse because of tightening, and more elasticity. Incontinence symptoms are eliminated or significantly reduced.

Changing the ratio of different types of collagen and elastin increases the mechanical properties, significantly altering the vaginal wall; specifically, it reduces its elasticity. Because the anterior vaginal wall acts as a support for the urethra and muscular lacunar tissue, loss of function leads to hypermobility of the urethra tissue and bladder neck, which manifests as stress urinary incontinence (stress from changes in intraabdominal pressure).

The use of laser energy leads to remodeling of the extracellular matrix and fibroblasts and activation of the vaginal tissue, improving the supporting properties of the vaginal wall. The increased elasticity in the vaginal wall is evaluated subjectively using a Visual Analog Scale and may not be assessed objectively.

References

1. Vizintin Z, Rivera M, Fistonić I, et al. Novel minimally invasive VSP Er:YAG laser treatments in gynecology. J Laser Health Acad 1:46, 2012.
2. Lee MS. Treatment of vaginal relaxation syndrome with an erbium:YAG laser using 90° and 360° scanning scopes: a pilot study & short-term results. Laser Ther 23:129, 2014.
3. Meijerink AM. Tissue composition of the vaginal wall in women with pelvic organ prolapse. Gynecol Obstet Invest 75:21, 2013.
4. Bezmenko AA, Schmidt AA, Koval AA, et al. Morphological substantiation of applying the Er:YAG laser for the treatment of stress urinary incontinence in women. J Obstet Women Dis 3:88, 2014.
5. Utian quality of life scale (UQOL). Available at *http://www.menopause.org/docs/default-document-library/uqol.pdf?sfvrsn=2.*

CREDITS

Chapter 1

Fig. 1-10   From Georgiou CA, Benatar M, Dumas P, et al. A cadaveric study of the arterial blood supply of the labia minora. Plast Reconstr Surg 136:167, 2015.

Chapter 3

Fig. 3-1   From Gorney M, Martello J. Patient selection criteria. Clin Plast Surg 26:37, 1999.

Chapter 4

Figs. 4-1, 4-3, 4-5, and 4-13   From Hamori CA. Postoperative clitoral hood deformity after labiaplasty. Aesthet Surg J 2013;33(7)1030-1036, by permission of Oxford University Press.

Figs. 4-4 and 4-8   From Hamori CA. Aesthetic surgery of the female genitalia: labiaplasty and beyond. Plast Reconstr Surg 134:661, 2014.

Chapter 14

Fig. 14-2   From Ostrzenski A. G-spot anatomy: a new discovery. J Sex Med 9:1355, 2012.

Chapter 17

Fig. 17-1   ©2016 Asclepion Laser Technologies, Jena–Germany. All rights reserved.

Figs. 17-2 and 17-3   Courtesy of University of Milano-Bicocca, San Gerardo Hospital, Monza, Italy - Department of Obstetrics and Gynecology, Chief Prof. Rodolfo Milani.

INDEX